STOP PREDICTING REVISIT LIFE

STOP PREDICTING REVISIT LIFE

Lessons from COVID-19

Vinay Sharma
Rabindranath Bhattacharyya
Sanjeev Kumar Mahajan
Himanshu Shekhar Mishra

BLOOMSBURY
NEW DELHI • LONDON • OXFORD • NEW YORK • SYDNEY

BLOOMSBURY INDIA
Bloomsbury Publishing India Pvt. Ltd
Second Floor, LSC Building No. 4, DDA Complex, Pocket C – 6 & 7,
Vasant Kunj, New Delhi 110070

BLOOMSBURY, BLOOMSBURY INDIA and the Diana logo
are trademarks of Bloomsbury Publishing Plc

First published in India 2022
This edition published 2022

ISBN: PB: 978-93-54350-92-4; e-Book: 978-93-54351-08-2
2 4 6 8 10 9 7 5 3 1

Typeset in Fournier MT Std by Manipal Technologies Limited
Printed and bound in India by Replika Press Pvt. Ltd.

To find out more about our authors and books, visit www.bloomsbury.com and sign
up for our newsletters

CONTENTS

1

Expect Everything–It's War

VINAY SHARMA
RABINDRANATH BHATTACHARYYA
SANJEEV KUMAR MAHAJAN
HIMANSHU SHEKHAR MISHRA

5 July 2021

Life has changed since the onset of the COVID-19 pandemic. COVID and vaccination have emerged as the keywords. Frontline workers are the saviours of the day, fighting the war relentlessly. India is going through one of the largest vaccination drives. Economic activities are slowly bouncing back. Power consumption is at its peak. The all-India peak electricity demand touched an all-time high of 191243 MW at 12:46 P.M. on 30 June 2021.[1] The worst-affected tourism and travel sector too is recovering, though tourists thronging popular tourist hotspots still pose a challenge for containing COVID-19. These are clear indicators of the revival of the Indian economy.

A couple of weeks back, the situation was completely different. '*Mujhe bacha lo*' (Please save me) was the final appeal of 38-year-old Raj Kumar Aggarwal to his colleagues. He was a corona warrior working in New Delhi's Lok Nayak Jai Prakash Hospital; he died due to COVID-19 on

29 April 2021.[2] The Indian Medical Association data shows that 747 doctors have died by the third week of April.[3] Officially, more than four lakh people have died in India due to COVID-19 till the first week of July 2021. At the same time, a little less than three crore people throughout India have also survived the pandemic.

For many children, the curtains came down on their childhood. The National Commission for Protection of Child Rights (NCPCR) informed the Supreme Court on 7 June 2021 that till then '26,176 children have lost a parent, 3,621 have been orphaned and 274 have been abandoned'.[4] People died gasping for oxygen. Dead bodies were floating in the rivers in lieu of a proper and dignified funeral. Lack of vaccines led to countless deaths among those in the 30–44 years age group. Conversely, many people miraculously survived even after a prolonged stay on artificial medical support. Limited effectiveness of therapy for COVID was evident everywhere. People were required to work, if not from office then from home. The hope is that someday people will be able to return to the pre-COVID life.

But this is the hope of people who hadn't suffered much. For those who have lost earning members of the family or those who are living a hand-to-mouth existence, the situation is pretty grim. On 30 June 2021, the Supreme Court directed 'the National Disaster Management Authority to recommend guidelines for ex gratia assistance on account of loss of life to the family members of the persons who died due to COVID-19'.[5] It is indeed a desired step. This will help the victims' families sustain themselves for some time before they can find a source of income and sustenance. But can any amount of money compensate for the loss of their near and dear ones? Can there be any compensation at all for death, more so for an untimely death? We are perplexed, confused and at a loss.

Since the beginning of the pandemic, leadership throughout the world has responded differently. A realistic expression of the loss and the best possible solutions have been the call of several nations. The impact of the pandemic is devastating. We lost so many of our near and dear ones. Hope, resilience and compassion were the need of the hour. Little did we realise in 2020 that the situation would be the same in 2021 as well. Some countries, which had been moving towards development, realised their compulsions and said, 'Let the virus do whatever it wants to', neither submitting to it nor caring about it. Nations began to need help so that they can navigate the rough sea with the least injury.

It seems that we are prisoners of time. The expression 'is it really happening?' has over a period of time turned into a question 'when would it go?' The shadow of the pandemic is stretching. This journey of pain, anguish and the presence of uncertainty has brought many lessons for us to remember and adopt. Some of us are agitated. Some of us are helpless. Survival takes precedence over everything else. Where does India stand? The answer is not simple. An all-in war is evident but have we taken notes? The learnings are being recorded by doctors, scientists, administrators, educationists, soldiers, businesses and farmers but not the common man. Whether we accept it or not, there are lessons of preparedness, life, togetherness, optimism, etc. Paradoxically, the word 'positive' has changed its meaning from something that signified the strength of a belief to something that now evokes fear and scorn. The word with such driving power has now suddenly took on a negative connotation. Alpha, Beta or Delta are not simply mathematical symbols. They are the symbols of COVID-19 variants, which could potentially turn society upside down at any moment. COVID-19 has invaded into our world of understanding.

It is clearly an extended war. The most important reconciliation creeping in throughout, whether we acknowledge it or not, is that analysis at any level is eliminating long-term prediction. It's not that we are losing hope. It's just that the importance of 'the present' has emphasised itself. People have a larger perspective on 'what they would do' and 'how things would be' after a few years from now, but that is largely associated with a hope that things would be as they were. Certainty with linearity has subdued.

Readers who read this text in the future might agree or might just wonder depending on the circumstances they will have faced and the narrative they will have heard. Despite that, an important lesson which will exist is that 'the testing times require wisdom at hand to be successful'. A predictive perspective might be the reflection of our desire to grow linearly in favourable times. This book describes the circumstances that persisted during COVID-19, which has traversed with devastating ease into 2020, 2021 and probably 2022, with a multangular point of view; it points out that whether one likes it or not, one should 'stop predicting and start living'.

By now, this may have started expressing itself as something which is coming out of an intense, frightful and stressful experience driven by misery all around. This may have started sounding like a sermon as well, which is known to everyone and we turn towards it in times of need and in such moments or era or period when our limitations do not allow us to meet challenges easily. We do not know the problems, leave aside the solutions. This book is about how predictive logic and models have been challenged within a very short span of time. It is not remedial and dialectic in approach but resonates a belief and rejuvenates a perspective of life which is enabled by living a life.

April of 2020, during one of our casual discussions, we realised that we are getting into a situation which is going to be pervasive and would have larger effects. Having spent a long time in different fields of learning, we entered into a discussion on 'what is happening?' This casual interaction amongst friends resulted in the need for a deeper understanding. The answers were diverse and full of surprises with every passing week. The element of surprise started carrying a feeling of devastation, pain, dismay, anguish and helplessness. Summer was approaching and all of us had plans to travel, which was diminishing day by day. The lockdown was getting extended and a large number of people were walking back home. Watching TV was not delightful. Just to mention, we were meeting and communicating through an online platform, which was the first thing that people did after being stuck in their homes.

The initial question traversed into the next phase: 'Why is this happening?' We had data to support our discussions though the multangular view was dominating. The next question 'what would happen?' emerged naturally, and we did not have answers. This was the time when this book came into existence. We had changed the draft twice till 4 November 2021, when India was celebrating Deepawali. The initial draft mentioned a progressive war, but we turned it into an ending war by December 2020 as the virus, in a disguise to retreat, was preparing for another battle. In February 2021, we declared the past 12 months as a period of the pandemic. By the time the book was reviewed, the chapters became redundant, and by 15 May 2021, we were rewriting several chapters. We had learnt the lesson 'stop predicting and start living'.

There is a lot in store. Let's get a glimpse of the areas of concern we have highlighted. There is so much that could have been added, but then we, as authors, have limitations. The chapter titled 'Indian Federalism: A Reality Check' reflects different provisions given in the Constitution of India. It discusses the institutional arrangements and the initiatives taken by the central and the state governments during the pandemic. It explains the history of development and livelihood in conjunction with the shielding and development of the environment. The Disaster Management Act, 2005, and the Epidemic Diseases (Amendment) Act, 2020, have laid down the mechanism to deal with these kind of situations. In order to make India disaster-resilient across all sectors, institutions like the National Disaster Management Authority play an important role. In this chapter, an attempt has been made to deal with the governance issues based on selected parameters.

The chapter titled 'Virus War: A Test of Leadership' talks about how COVID-19 has challenged the whole of human race and has tested leadership at all levels with all its characteristics. An enemy with an immense capacity of multiplication with mutation suddenly hit the globe. Fortresses of algorithms beaming with the confidence of tested models could not bear the blow. The virus entered forcefully, compelling decision makers to fight. A direction was needed and directives were required. Individual, group, community and mass tendencies came into play simultaneously. The response of the leadership was a reflection of whatever happened at different levels. The quality of a leadership is proven when it is tested. We always expect leadership to be ideal and expect all the unexpected. But the unexpected happens not simply because of the failure of the leadership; it happens also because of the unpreparedness of the community and its resistance to be prepared. Then the basic duty of the leadership is to prepare the community for the unexpected and to train them for behaving in a responsible manner in the worst of times. This brings us to the concept of Ram Rajya in the Gandhian sense. Mahatma Gandhi said, 'By Ramarajya I do not mean Hindu Raj. I mean by Ramarajya Divine Raj, the Kingdom of God. For me Rama and Rahim are one and the same deity. I acknowledge no other God but the one God of truth and righteousness.' He further said (and it is quoted from the same source) that 'the highest form of freedom carries with it the greatest measure of discipline and humility'. He has elaborated upon the responsibilities and duties of people towards each other alongwith mutual respect, love and compassion.[6] Goswami Tulsidasji in a quatrain verse in *Shri Ramcharitmanas*[7] has written:

दैहिक दैविक भौतिक तापा। राम राज नहिं काहुहि ब्यापा॥
सब नर करहिं परस्पर प्रीती। चलहिं स्वधर्म निरत श्रुति नीती॥

> In the whole of Sri Rama's dominions there was none who suffered from the affliction of any kind—whether of the body, or proceeding from divine or supernatural agencies or that caused by another living being. All men loved one another: each followed one's prescribed duty, conformably to the precepts of the Vedas. Uttar Kaand; Chaupai- 20, Line 1.

The next chapter, 'Pandemic Narrative and the Mindset of Civil Society', focuses on the behavioural pattern of civil society that changed to a great extent by the sudden emergence and development of a pandemic. Whether it was the plague, which emerged in Athens in 430 BC or the Spanish flu of 1918 or the current COVID pandemic, human history has shown time and again that the third sector of society, belonging neither to the public nor the private sector, responded in an unpredictable manner. The predictable anxieties of civil society suddenly became unpredictable, and the state–civil society relationships became fraught with these stresses. Would they be able to enjoy the erstwhile guaranteed civil and economic rights?

In the pandemic, the government dealt with various issues in a novel way, which led to a few questions. Did those decisions meant for collective good take into consideration human rights? What were the specific features of the response strategy of the people? What was the specific entertainment narrative of the pandemic? How did the political society of Bihar and the USA behave alike? We have explored all these issues by comparing them to the plague epidemic of 430 BC and the Spanish flu pandemic of 1918.

The COVID crisis marks a watershed moment in the recent history of the Indian media. The pandemic saw the first attempt at institutionalising a crisis communication protocol at the national level. With newspapers unable to print, millions of viewers switched to their TV sets to get first-hand information on the pandemic and its debilitating impact on the Indian economy and society. Based on the author's experience of gathering news since the first day of the imposition of the lockdown, especially his ground reports, the data collected and his analyses as a field correspondent, the chapter called 'COVID-19 and the Challenge of Crisis Communication' delineates the problems reporters faced. It narrates how TV news journalists had to reformat their conventional newsgathering techniques and television equipment and accessories to protect themselves and their crew while reporting. We further faced complex moral and ethical questions in terms of what to report and what not to.

More importantly, this chapter highlights the urgent need to develop and codify a crisis communication protocol. We argue that the dissemination of credible information during a public health disaster is directly related to the freedom and access journalists are given. It is also important to protect the rights of the media and ensure that the newsgathering process is not restricted. Attempts to 'condition' can distort the natural news flow, which is critical in such a crisis situation.

This pandemic has exposed the weaknesses in the existing public health communication systems. In this age of globalisation of news and information, developed countries like the United States, Britain and Italy failed to employ viable emergency measures to sensitise and alert their citizens to the dangers posed by the outbreak of COVID in China. This raises fundamental questions about the efficacy of crisis communication systems that were functional there. In this context, the chapter highlights the need to develop a blueprint of outbreak risk communication protocol to fight such public health exigencies in future.

The chapter argues that it is important for a populous country like India to strictly implement the goals enshrined in The Sendai Framework for Disaster Risk Reduction 2015–2030, which specifically outlines an urgent need to develop disaster risk reduction communication policies to disseminate a culture of prevention and strengthen community involvement in public education campaigns.

The chapter 'Agriculture in the Time of COVID-19: A Beacon of Hope' largely delineates the broader impact the pandemic has had on India's farm sector. The chapter is based on interviews with important stakeholders, including Union Agriculture Minister

Narendra Singh Tomar and the late Union Consumer Affairs, Food and Public Distribution Minister Ram Vilas Paswan at the height of the crisis in India, data accessed from the agriculture ministry, the food ministry, the finance ministry and the home ministry of the Government of India, Prime Minister's Office, debates in the Parliament and important reports of the Census Commission of India. The chapter attempts to deconstruct the comparative impact of the pandemic on crucial sectors and highlights how agriculture provided strength to India's fight against COVID. As the RBI governor publicly pointed out during the crisis, agriculture emerged as 'a sliver of brightness amidst the encircling gloom'.[8]

The chapter also studies the 1918 Spanish flu, which was accompanied by a weak monsoon, that had wreaked havoc on India's agriculture sector. More than a hundred years ago, the famine-like situation in parts of India had led to forced migration from rural areas to urban centres, which turned out to be catastrophic for the whole country. Around 17 million Indians died during the Spanish flu. This was in stark contrast to COVID, which was accompanied by an above-normal monsoon. Also, the corona crisis witnessed a different kind of migration—this time by millions of workers from urban industrial centres going back to their homes in rural India.

The next chapter, 'Migrant Workers and Food Security during the Pandemic: An Acid Test for Government Policies', focuses on the biggest saga of reverse interstate migration during the nationwide lockdown that was announced on short notice. The saga revealed the wretched and marginalised conditions of migrant labourers, especially with respect to food security. A large part of India assumed that these labourers were carriers of COVID and were unwelcome in their own villages. This chapter focuses on the reasons for such reverse migration and the policy changes that are required to avoid such incidents in the future.

The chapter, on the basis of a plethora of events reported in the newspapers, news blogs and news webs, analyses government data as well as that of non-government organisations related to the United Nations, focusing on the socio-economic status of migrant workers in India. From thereon, the chapter goes on to discuss the appalling food security situation owing to the inefficient public distribution system.

The chapter titled 'Unpredictable Lives and Livelihood with COVID-19' reflects how the pandemic has led to far-reaching social and economic imbalances in India. This situation has provided an opportunity to assess the strengths and deficiencies of governments at the national and state levels. The government was not fully prepared to face the consequences at the start of the pandemic, in terms of a national cohesive strategy to combat its possible devastating impact on human health and economy. Every individual in India was affected because of the nationwide lockdown. It had a debilitating impact on economic activities as it led to a severe disruption of business activities leading to an unprecedented employment crisis. As the number of COVID patients rose alarmingly in India, the health infrastructure became incapable of handling the numbers. This unprecedented crisis pushed millions of families into acute financial crisis. This also led to a significant rise in reports of domestic violence. To overcome these problems, the Government of India announced[9] a series of relief and fiscal stimulus measures worth nearly ₹20 lakh crore.

The role of educationists and education had been to facilitate the whole narrative of living. When humans started getting confident about controlling things, they realised that they should direct all the learnings towards profit and benefit, and then they started utilising humans as a resource. The result was that the whole of the education system directed its attention to train people rather than to make them learn and leave them independently to choose between alternatives. It was structurally decided about which kind of people would do what in their lives, how they would do that and this is how the whole narrative was created. The outcomes were measured in terms of the role they would play and the compensation they would get. These were the only two measurement criteria which have been existing for the past 4–5 decades. The world invariably kept following that; education and educationists started focusing on the benchmark model and kept incrementally complimenting it, whenever necessary.

The chapter called 'Education for Education' suggests that things are changing—policies are being reconstituted and revisited and are being honestly and dedicatedly implemented. It's time that educationists also revisit their roles and know how to do them.

In the concluding chapter, 'Towards a Post COVID-19 World', the authors note that the world must realise that preparation and preparedness is the key which can only come with resilience and togetherness. In a post-COVID India, we look for a society where there will be a doctor in every 200 households. We wish that the economy and society will be supportive of farmers and not just farms. Education will be willing to revisit its orientation, process, pedagogy and output every now and then and will keep everyone near to their roots. This will enhance versatility and multiplicity, not extreme specialisation. Leadership will percolate down to the grassroots level in its entirety and strength, reducing a need for predictability. Policies and market development will lead to prosperity and not just demand. Economic measurements will remain a guiding force and not the only driving force. The market opportunity will enhance the opportunity for participation for all and not opportunism. The COVID-19 pandemic has exposed fundamental weaknesses in the existing governance architecture at the global level. The world had faith in predictions but the pandemic led to unpredictability. It is evident from the beginning of the coronavirus pandemic. No one has been sure about when the second wave will culminate to the third and the fourth. The scientists, epidemiologists, virologists and researchers are struggling hard to predict the outcome of the pandemic. Hence, each one of us has been forced to live in uncertainty. The manner in which the world's most powerful countries with the most advanced healthcare infrastructure collapsed has raised critical questions about the state of preparedness of the global community to fight such public health disasters in future. The global community must address the critical questions that have arisen in the wake of the pandemic and take urgent cooperative steps to address them. The world must learn the lessons posed by the COVID-19 pandemic. The lessons of Spanish flu of 1918 were largely ignored, which aggravated the crisis more than hundred years later. All of us who have faced death, loss, anxiety, pain and anguish would be able to understand what people have experienced and would never like to imagine this pandemic coming back. Though everyone wishes to get it over with as soon as they possibly can and to never think of it, we should not refrain from leaving lessons behind. Lessons not only on 'if it happens' but also on 'why it may not happen'.

The global community cannot afford to make the same mistake again. Let's stop predicting and start living—living together.

Our book reflects on the first 18 months of the COVID pandemic period, starting with the first COVID-19 case reported in Kerala on 30 January 2020 till the decline of the second COVID-19 wave in July 2021. As this book goes for publication, India is in the midst of coping with Omicron, a new variant of COVID (B.1.1.529), designated as a 'variant of concern' by WHO on 26 November 2021. As of 12 December 2021, a total of 36 confirmed cases of Omicron have been reported in India and this 'highly transmissible' Omicron variant has spread to at least 59 nations.

2

Indian Federalism

A Reality Check

SANJEEV KUMAR MAHAJAN

Biological debacles occur due to the wrath of nature, mishaps, human blunders or intentional activities of anti-state agencies. Natural catastrophes could include pandemics, leading to many deaths and bringing people down to their knees. However, during the COVID-19 pandemic, inevitable cracks appeared in India's federalism. It was a reflection of its changing face at the beginning of the pandemic. Several differences between the centre and the state governments emerged. Centre-state cooperative federalism's fissures raised fundamental issues that need to be addressed now as the pandemic rages through the country. It is imperative that states act as the first line of defense against the crisis; their stand is equally significant. It is interesting to note that new dimensions of challenges emerged during both the waves of the pandemic. The compelling controversies related to centre-state relations during the pandemic are discussed for both waves separately in this chapter.

A pandemic reflects the global outbreak of a disease. It was initially classified as an epidemic that spread at a faster speed across regional and global boundaries. A pandemic can be caused by influenza or other viruses. However, once in a while, a new virus surfaces that does not behave as anticipated. That is when a pandemic breaks out because individuals do not have susceptibility to the new infection.[1]

There have been several virulent viruses that have left their mark. However, the most dangerous one recorded in history was the Spanish flu of 1918. It was presumed that this virus infected one-third of the world. After more than a century, the world is once again in the grip of a new virus named COVID-19 or novel coronavirus disease. It was recognised as a public health emergency on 30 January 2020.

The global timeline of the outbreak of the COVID-19 crisis is seen below:

Figure 2.1: Global Timeline

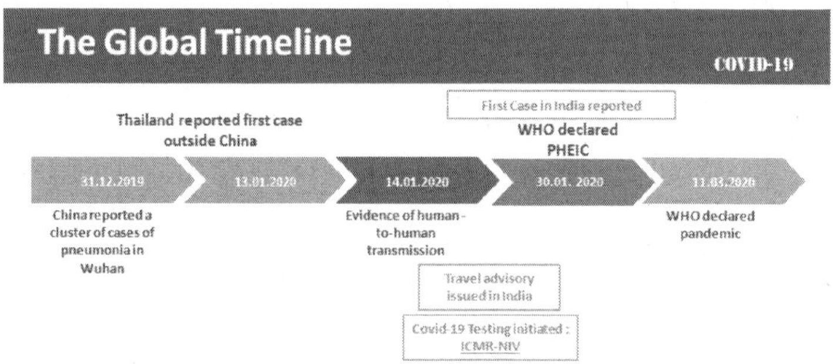

Source: Departmental Related Parliamentary Standing Committee (21 December 2020). 229th Report on Management of COVID-19 Pandemic and Related Issues, Rajya Sabha Secretariat. New Delhi. Page 1

The World Health Organization suggested that countries take immediate action to treat, detect and lower transmission of the virus to save lives. Realising the gravity of the situation, the pandemic was declared a 'notified disaster'[2] by the Government of India. Disasters, as defined by the UN, refer to a 'serious disruption of the functioning of the community or society involving widespread human, material, economic and environmental losses and impacts, which exceed the ability of the affected community or society to cope up using its resources'.[3] The reason for the government to pronounce COVID as a disaster was to facilitate funding to provide assistance to the affected victims in combating the pandemic. In the second wave, India had to change the strategy to control the numbers of COVID-affected patients. In his review meeting on 9 April 2021 with state chief ministers and the representatives of the union territories, the Prime Minister of India gave a new mantra of 'Test, Trace and Treat'.

Federalism in Times of a Pandemic

Federalism in India is a debatable issue. While some people call it 'quasi-federal', 'competitive federalism', or 'cooperative federalism', the bigger debate underlying is whether India is a federal State.[4] It implies that national, state and local governments have an interactive relationship rather than individual policies.

The Indian constitution has a quasi-federal structure mentioned initially in the Government of India Act, 1935. The Act highlighted and emphasised cooperation between the centre and states to achieve directed socio-economic growth. Apart from this, the framers of the

Indian constitution relied on the experiences of the federations of the United States of America, Canada and Australia regarding the problems they faced in maintaining their federation structures. Hence, the measures to resolve the problem areas faced by these countries were taken into consideration while framing the Indian constitution.

History suggested a need for a stronger centre. Indian federalism was designed to be flexible, and a provision was created to temporarily enhance the centre's power temporarily, should a situation so warrant. Overall, the strength of the centre lies in its legislative, administrative and financial powers. It allows the centre to take control of the state legislation and administration in extraordinary situations. India has a federal structure of governance, where the union and state governments have legislative, executive and judicial powers. It has differentiated the jurisdiction, powers and functions performed by the union and the state governments.

The powers and role of the centre in legislative, administrative and financial relations have been explicitly mentioned in the Indian constitution. Under the constitution, the union government has been given authority over the states to ascertain the unity and integrity of the nation. Thus, the Constitution of India provides for a set of rules through which the country is to be ruled by the elected government. On the other hand, constitutionalism reflects governance; it's about respecting its citizens' individual and collective rights. Hence, it can well be argued that the Indian constitution creates a model of cooperative federalism. This point can further be understood by discussing a few essential provisions mentioned in the constitution.

The following provisions highlight the centre-state cooperation:

The Seventh Schedule elucidates and enumerates allocations of powers and functions between the centre and the states by outlining the tasks carried out under the centre, state and concurrent lists. It means that the lower-level unit of government has been empowered to make decisions concerning matters mentioned in the state list. There are 52 (originally 47) items under the concurrent list. There is an exception to the constitution's rule that the central law will prevail in case of conflict on any law subject.

The All India Service: The judicial system in India oversees the implementation of the central and state laws with the help of the All India Service.[5]

Coordination between the union and the states: Article 263 of the Indian constitution provides an interstate council. This council aims to follow a calculative and systematised approach to achieve the comprehensive socio-economic advancement of all sections of society.

How Has Indian Federalism Faired in Governance of COVID-19?

Indian democracy has been tested several times since Independence. Each time, it was successful in dealing with the challenges it faced. For example, the annual budgetary processes at the central and state governments are now independent exercises and must pass through the Parliament and the respective state legislatures. Further, the Finance Commission was established under Article 280 of the constitution to define the financial relations between the centre and states and review them every five years. These commonalities have helped the federal structure to strengthen federalism in India. However, no one had probably perceived facing a predicament such as this pandemic. It has taken the world by surprise, and India is no exception.

The pandemic has ruthlessly destroyed the economies of both developed and developing nations. It is a testing time for Indian federalism too. The world waited with bated breath for vaccines to arrive. It is understood that while they are not the magic formula, they are still a ray of hope. The mantra, therefore, has been: Stop predicting and focus on managing the pandemic.

The pandemic has been a litmus test for flexible, coherent, efficient and effective decision-making processes and their capability to meet the rising challenges. Strong and cogent leadership at the central and state levels was evident because many states announced lockdown and sealed their borders even before the union government imposed a complete lockdown for 21 days to control the spread of the virus on 24 March 2020.

With this background, a critical assessment has been done based on the selected parameters. The first wave had some grave controversies, which are:

Breach of cooperative federalism: Earlier in the chapter, it was mentioned that the powers and functions have been demarcated between the centre and the states to maintain the concept of cooperative federalism. However, the stress is on having an efficient and effective health infrastructure and sanitation during the pandemic. This area falls solely under the domain of the states. However, under Section 35(1), the Government of India unilaterally implemented and invoked the Disaster Management Act, 2005, in the entire country without consulting the states. Through another provision under Section 35(2)(1), it is proposed that 'coordination of actions of Ministry or Departments of the Government of India, state governments, national authority, state authorities, governmental and non-governmental organisations concerning disaster management shall be consulted in case of a disaster'. However, the central government did not consult the states before implementing the national lockdown. Thus, the selective application of the Disaster Management Act, 2005, created fissures in Indian federalism.

Trust deficit in leadership: Many review meetings on the COVID situation in the country were conducted and chaired by the prime minister and attended by all chief ministers. It was evident from the outcome of these meetings that some states did not appear to be fully in sync with the policies of the centre to control the pandemic. For example, the question of zone classification into red, orange and green drew unexpected criticism from a number of states. The states believed that public health and sanitation was a state subject and they knew best about the challenges they were facing. The Disaster Management Act of 2005 also refers to having a 'national plan' under Section

11 and issues a mandatory instruction under Section 6(2) by the centre to the states. However, Section 11(2) endorses that the national plan can only be formulated after consultation with the states.

Furthermore, the migrant crisis also brought up a lack of effective leadership in handling the movement of the migrants. Both the centre and the states failed to visualise and formulate a comprehensive plan to avoid the migrant crisis in these difficult times, which aggravated the spread of the virus. So, during these desperate times, a trust deficit in leadership emerged. However, Microsoft's fellow benefactor Bill Gates and WHO have praised Indian Prime Minister Narendra Modi for dealing with the COVID flare-up in India and the evaluation taken to contain the spread of the lethal infection. Gates also appreciated the government for using innovative tools such as the Aarogya Setu app to track and trace infected people.

Unavailability of funds with the states: The pandemic has forced the centre and the states to impose periodic lockdowns. This has resulted in a total halt of economic activities, leading to a complete collapse of the revenue stream. Even during the unlock period, states could not generate revenue because the supply chain was disrupted. The significant sources of revenue for the conditions are liquor sales, stamp duty from land/ property transactions and duty on petroleum products. As a result, economic activities have not resumed or gone back to pre-pandemic levels. This has aggravated the precarious financial position because it has resulted in the loss of state goods and service tax collection. On the other hand, the liabilities for carrying out welfare schemes, interest on borrowings and salaries to employees have remained the same even during these testing times. This has made the states heavily dependent on the centre for financial support.

Further, the unilateral decision of the Government of India to suspend the Members of Parliament Local Area Development Scheme funds stopped the inflow of resources to the states. The central government's move to divert funds from the Consolidated Fund of India without consulting the states also fractured the concept of cooperative federalism. These extraordinary situations can only be dealt with effectively if an adequate supply of funds and necessary equipment are made available by the centre since the states are the first responders of the pandemic. The centre has to respond to the needs of the individual states to strengthen their health infrastructure, rather than make the states dependent.

The muddle of corporate social responsibility: Modern corporate enterprises exert considerable influence on civil society, polity and a nation's economy by embracing efforts to improve the community.[6] It is pertinent to understand the responsibility of the individual enterprise to meet its social obligations towards society. The Companies Act, 2013, lays down the rules for incorporating a company, responsibilities of the company and its directors and the method of its dissolution.

Section 135 of the Companies Act, 2013, states that the concept of corporate social responsibility (CSR), which implies a compulsory benefaction for the large enterprises having a net worth of more than ₹5 billion

(₹500 crore) or a turnover of more than ₹10 billion (₹1,000 crore) or a net profit of more than ₹50 million (₹5 crore), requires companies to pay out a minimum of 2 per cent of its annual profit towards activities mentioned in the Seventh Schedule of the Act. The Ministry of Corporate Affairs vide General Circular No.15/2020 dated 10 April 2020 issued COVID-related frequently asked questions on CSR.[7] It is clear from the document that contributions made towards Prime Minister's Citizen Assistance and Relief in Emergency Situations (PM CARES) Fund shall qualify as CSR expenditure, vide item No. (viii) of the Schedule VII of the Companies Act, 2013. Apart from this, any amount spent on COVID-related activities shall also qualify as CSR expenditure.

However, the contribution made to the Chief Minister's Relief Fund or State Relief Fund for COVID was not included in Schedule VII of the Companies Act, 2013. Hence, any contribution of funds there does not qualify as permissible CSR expenditure. Therefore, the only donations made to State Disaster Management Authorities (SDMA) under Item XII of Schedule VII qualify as CSR expenditure.

It can be concluded that the GoI has deliberately dissuaded these enterprises from making any contribution to relief measures undertaken by the state governments. Therefore, there is a sense that the central government wants the states to be financially dependent for managing the pandemic.

India is continuing its battle against the second wave of coronavirus pandemic, necessitating new dimensions of policy defiance between the centre and the state governments.

The realm of federal beliefs has been hit hard because of a political scuffle over crucial matters related to controlling the pandemic.

Fissures in India's COVID vaccine policy: India's minister of health and family welfare announced way back in October 2020 that the GoI is likely to receive 400–500 million vaccine doses to cover about 200–300 million people by the end of March 2021. Accordingly, the national COVID strategy was evolved to vaccinate people in three phases. The first phase, which started on 16 January 2021, laid stress on vaccinating health and frontline workers. The second phase, initiated on 1 March 2021, was divided into two parts. In the first part, individuals above 60 years with specific comorbidities were included in the vaccination priority list. GoI soon expanded the ambit to include everyone above the age of 45 years. In addition, during the thick of elections in five states, the GoI announced that everyone above the age of 18 would be vaccinated.

The controversy over vaccination started in the third phase. The central government solely carried out the first two phases of the vaccination programme. The GoI was exclusively responsible for the procurement and distribution of the vaccine among the states. The trouble started when chief ministers of a few states demanded decentralisation of the vaccine initiative.

The situation was aggravated after the release of 'Liberalized Pricing and Accelerated National COVID-19 Vaccination Strategy' by GoI. It contained the provision that 50 per cent of vaccine doses manufactured by Indian pharmaceuticals will be supplied to GoI at an agreed price. The remaining were provided to states, private hospitals and the corporate/industry at a negotiated price. The states cried foul over the pricing differentials. First, the GoI was criticised, especially by different opposition-ruled states. Second, Indian vaccine manufacturers could not produce doses per the states' requirements and the shortage of supply was inexcusable. Hence, the unbalanced acquisition of vaccines widened the rift between the centre and state governments.

Another issue that the states faced was the complex structure of procuring immunisation from foreign vaccine manufacturers. The latter refused to negotiate with the states and preferred to do so with the centre only. The centre finally decided to procure 75 per cent of vaccines for the states and started distributing them throughout the country from 21 June 2021 onwards. Lastly, how to fund the procurement of vaccines remains a million-dollar question. Indian states faced a financial crunch as most economic activities have remained suspended for quite some time. Ultimately, the GoI decided on centralised procurement and distribution of vaccine. The latest decision of the GoI, while writing this book, is that all eligible people will be inoculated by the end of 2021. This will be a litmus test, as the whole world is watching India's vaccine progress.

Judicial governance: Centre-state relations and interstate relations in India have seen ups and downs since Independence. Lack of agreement during India's biggest humanitarian crisis since Independence has resulted in judicial activism. It is well argued that the judiciary is bound to protect individual rights.

We have witnessed numerous situations like migrants returning to their homes on foot in the absence of public transport during the first wave of the pandemic. Recently, political rallies organised in different poll-bound states and religious congregations held by various sections of society at the beginning of 2021 have been significant causes for the surge in cases. Pressure on the health infrastructure, life-saving drugs and oxygen availability during the second wave are examples of the judiciary attacking the institutions responsible for controlling the pandemic. The Madras High Court has used the very harsh word—'murderers'—against the Election Commission of India and blamed it for spreading COVID. The Delhi High Court also made similar remarks while exercising judicial review and cognisance of lawsuits related to allocating and distributing oxygen and life-saving drugs. Many private hospitals had to approach the high court to seek its involvement in passing instructions to the concerned agencies to supply oxygen to protect the lives of individuals under Section 21 of the Indian constitution.

The Delhi High Court observed that it is difficult for the legislature and the executives to accept their failures in handling the pandemic. The crisis has forced the judiciary to overstep their role and transform themselves into an agency of judicial governance.

Interstate relations during the pandemic: The situations where centre-state relations became strained have been discussed earlier. There are quite a few examples where the absence of cooperation between the states can be seen during both waves. The dispute between the states of Karnataka and Kerala over the sealing of borders along the national highways was one of them. The judiciary had to intervene to ensure vehicular movement regarding healthcare on the national highways passing through these states.

The National Human Rights Commission recently had to issue notices to the union jal sakti ministry and states of Uttar Pradesh and Bihar after receiving complaints of dead bodies floating in the Ganges. Both the states accused each other of dumping dead bodies to show lower mortality rates. Even the international community raised an alarm regarding inaccurate data. It has been reported that the high death rate during the second wave overburdened funeral and burial grounds across the country, which is one reason why dead bodies were disposed of in the Ganges. That could also have been because of faith-related issues or simply wanting to avoid infection from dead bodies. Ultimately, it is the failure of the states to not create enough awareness against superstitions. The inadequacy of the executive has resulted in the judiciary taking day-to-day control of pandemic-related solutions. The government reacted a bit too late, costing human lives and dignity, rather than being proactive in its approach. Is it a cover-up? We will know soon if and when the investigations go through and the guilty are punished.

Learning to Be in It Together

Governance challenges in these times of the pandemic are many and varied. The situation is quite fluid, and the government is found grappling with changing conditions every day. The prime reason for that is the world has not faced a pandemic for a century, and no one knows a sure way of dealing with it.

The concept of cooperative federalism has been under attack when it comes to the governance of the COVID crisis. On the other hand, the states supported the centre in the imposition of lockdown throughout last year. In 2021, the GoI left the decision of lockdown to individual states after keeping in mind local conditions. It remains to be seen how this extreme form of decentralisation with only guidelines from the centre will work out in the end. The US also decentralised similarly, and that left citizens and the authorities in confusion and chaos. In India, people do not know which region is closed and which is open to conduct their business. The manufacturing community has been allowed to go on, but transportation is affected. Buyers are demotivated to carry on in this atmosphere of uncertainty and confusion. There has to be a proper balance between centralisation and decentralisation to get effective results, which are basic public administration principles.

Challenges are many, and the need of the hour is to find solutions for self-reliance, strengthen civil society and increase manufacturing to deal with a dwindling economy. To enhance the capabilities and capacity of the states, the centre must treat states as equal, and everyone should work in collaboration to overcome this crisis.

This brings us to a positive impact that India sees—communities and NGOs coming together in this hour of need. People across the country have organised community kitchens to distribute free food to the needy. Ensuring adequate supply of oxygen, medicines and arranging beds for the deprived section of society are being done on social media.

While this is heart-warming to witness, we wonder if the government has failed its citizens or if the crisis is so humungous that it is unable to cope. The government always seems to be catching up rather than being proactive. When it has been proactive, problems have invariably been resolved. Some hospitals set up expressly to fight COVID hired doctors for an eight-hour shift at ₹6,000 in Delhi. After a couple of days, they were fired via WhatsApp, stating that their services were unnecessary. These doctors had complained about the lack of facilities for doctors, such as sub-standard personal protective equipment (PPE) kits, the same area for donning and doffing the kits—a lethal mixture for spreading the virus—and many such instances. This shows that even though the government aims to be prepared for the next wave, the ground reality does not reflect this.

There are many lessons to learn, but petty politics over the government's actions seems to be the primary focus rather than the problem at hand. These issues remain elusive because politicians are unwilling to change their ways, and the common man suffers.

3

Virus War

A Test of Leadership

VINAY SHARMA

An enemy with an immense capacity of multiplication with mutation suddenly hit the globe. Fortresses of algorithms beaming with the confidence of tested models could not bear the blow. COVID-19 entered forcefully, compelling decision-makers to fight. Leadership was challenged at all the levels with all its characteristics. Direction was needed and directives were required. Individual, group, community and mass tendencies came into play simultaneously. The response of the leadership was the reflection of whatever happened at different levels.

Let's Start from the Beginning

Let's try to go back to early 2020, when news started flowing about the possible spread of the virus. International travel was at its peak. The festival of Holi in India was approaching and thousands of travelers were inbound, though that was not the only reason. Strict protocol, statements, guidelines and advice were coming from all quarters, especially from organisations and institutions which had a clue of the situation and could somehow apprehend the times to come. The information specifically was flowing from the organisations which were feeling responsible for the situation. The call was to move away from places that were experiencing the initial spread. Individually one was unable to imagine, analyse and was not even afraid. People sitting with their families were worried not knowing what to do and not having even a slightest clue that perhaps many would be losing their loved ones unimaginably soon. After much debate, collective wisdom prevailed and the immediate response was to find the origin and the culprit. But where was COVID-19? What would one do as and when it appears? The world is so entangled or globalised, so to say, that aware intelligentsia through their institutions were unable to muster strength and find a way of buying the words 'Let's stop'. The world has been nurturing hierarchy, and we were all looking upto someone to give a timeline and direction because that is what we have been doing. We have been 'predicting'.

The virus started spreading. Medical science and the sciences came forward first. Their leadership took a stand, entered the virus war and created protocol. There was a free flow of information. The entire value chain got repulsively instigated. Prevention kits, serving equipment, supplies, remedies, medicines and an intense concentration on the development of vaccines came into being. Somehow, the supply of oxygen got overlooked.

Community-level decision-making was required and was being exemplified even by some of the nations. The response was 'defence'. Lessons were learnt. Broader guidelines, data, protocol and related results were indicative of what to do. Community and community-based political leadership was looked upon. Decisions were taken. Bhutan, New Zealand and several other countries, on the one hand, and tribal communities of the Indian Ocean and the Himalayas, on the other, became examples. But predictive methodology and an insight was still prominent and the time of elimination of the enemy was being impatiently calculated. Probably, this is what the virus was asking for, as that calculation prompted its mutation. This should not be taken in a literal sense and it might not have something to do with the timing of the scientific progression of the virus, but remember that we are discussing an enemy and we wish to imagine its intelligence.

An interesting scenario was evolving, that though the virus had a travel history, it had reached almost everywhere; we thought that it would stagnate its growth and since we have partially submitted to it by locking down everything, it would subside. Meanwhile, the pharmaceutical and research and development leadership got committed to develop, produce and disburse the vaccine which was predicted as a negotiated midpoint between the virus and the political and economic leadership. Everything seemed right. The political leadership all around the world started preparing for the 'unlock'. Different scenarios came up in different countries. Only a few could see early devastation and death through unprecedented spread. Here, mass tendency played a typical role wherein the world realised that due to a specific flow of economic progression leading to mutually decided growth parameters, density and interdependencies of people reached to a point of no return. As if the enemy knew and understood it well. Despite the differentiated travel history of the virus, response time and resource capability of the medical, academic and research and development leaderships, their response mechanism was similar, which was lock, test, isolate, partially unlock, vaccinate and win.

The initial loss of some of the nations, especially in terms of death, was empathised by some. Several debates on the virus being universal in its outlook towards developed and developing nations came up. Many seemingly successful nations while being cautious started wondering on climatic and other conditions, immunity levels and other factors, which could have potentially saved them. Remember, predictive nature cannot be changed overnight and has always been there.

The masses had different levels of reception in different regions. At some places, they followed the regulations about wearing a mask, social distancing and staying at home, whereas at other places they responded according to their convenience and largely did not follow the norms. The police leadership let their force into the war strongly and admirably while supporting the medical warriors. Ambulatory services, nursing and support teams and several others who challenged their physical limitations and sacrificed their family lives to save and serve others were admired, but were not sympathised by the masses for their efforts; otherwise they would have shown greater restraint and concern. Does it imply that the masses do not listen to anyone? Does it mean that individuals worry, groups discuss, communities manage and fight and the masses don't care?

The executive leadership at the government and corporate levels was collecting and analysing information while planning and executing the process of locking and unlocking. Their awareness has been strong as they have had access to the requisite data and information. Their insight led them to a major question of 'how and when'. Answers were being found.

Economic leadership along with the executive had already analysed the losses as they had models. Plans and processes were being rolled out. Although traversing through similar processes and predictive modeling, different results were being reported from different nations, but there has always been a scope of increasing, decreasing, intensifying and diluting the factors in the models. Therefore, when some countries reported a second wave and compulsive lockdowns, many reanalysed their respective paths and found those to be reliable. This is not a wrong approach because it has been tested for decades, but was it really working?

End of the Pandemic Was Projected

The end of the pandemic was predicted. We as authors also discussed the last phase of expressions. Only a few could have known that predicting the unpredictable could be an entrapment. There were alarm bells, but we wanted to get out of the situation. The compulsion of running the economies and nations was overwhelming. Dates and calendars were staring into our faces. Cost-benefit analysis was becoming prominent while emphasising its directive power.

We started finalising the text. Wrote the introduction and conclusion; finally declared victory on 15 February 2021, living a full circle of belief and disbelief starting from around 15 February 2020. There was a sigh of relief when we sent the chapters for review. Vaccination started and phases were meticulously planned. The economy was unlocked and workers started going back. Students started going back to schools and colleges. Campuses were reopened. The boarders were invited through the protocol of quarantine. Meanwhile, COVID-19 deceptively made us believe that it has lost the ground. The sale of masks was reported at an all-time low. Hotels, restaurants and tourism were back on their feet, overcrowding places. It was celebration time. Growth and rejuvenation became the points of concentration.

COVID-19 Sprung Back as COVID-19 in 2021

We were expecting an edited version of the book. Only four weeks later, by the 1st anniversary of the first lockdown, a mutant COVID, feeling hurt by the response of mankind, not only to its might but also to the lessons it made us learn, came back in full force rapidly multiplying and taking the number of cases to an all-time high. Leadership at all levels was compelled to retrieve all the steps except for corona warriors.

One and all panicked due to this unprecedented and devastating blow. Almost everyone was touched somehow. Political and executive leadership could not immediately get out of the processes they initiated in terms of rejuvenation. All the others were engaged in pulling up the scenario in their own terms.

Only medical leadership was in a continued war because they could not think of anything else and they were the most hard-pressed.

This time the enemy was after the breathing system of the infected. It was cutting the lifeline as if it knew that the backup of this lifeline will fall short of supplies. It was aware of the doctor-patient and the hospital bed-patient ratios. The most elites of the elites could also not arrange for hospital beds and oxygen supply. Did we ever imagine that a dead organism had a strategy or a survival plan, which could hit the enabled, developed world, unaware of its weak spots and that too with an intensity and a speed which was never imagined?

The first review of the chapters reflected a perplexed prospective readership. The scenario which seemed to be under control had completely changed over a period of time. The first draft was away from reality.

The War Still Had a Long Way to Go

It took us sometime to revisit the whole thing. Though the expression of a warrior leadership which I wanted to extend was still true but had to be revisited with a scene of a war still aggressively to be fought and far from victory, which I declared earlier. This raised a pertinent question. What would the leadership do? What should the leadership be when a winning war is required to be fought again? Resources in short supply, human resource motivated, though anticipating an the end. Major questions which came to the fore now were: How to tell people to stop once again and till when? How to convince people to do what should be done? How to change or divert the narrative from individual growth to resilience and contentment? How to change the growth parameters, benchmarks and measurement scales? Leadership is about creating precedence, not about following it. History would discuss this war as it has been doing as ever. Standard operating procedures and protocol would be the lessons, but the actual need of the future generation would be to pick up scales and benchmarks of decision-making, courage and bringing out people safely.

Just to remind you before going ahead that this is not a discussion about leaders; it is all about leadership. I urge you not to imagine faces, even though instinctively one would be tempted to do so.

Non-Denial Is the Key

You must have heard the famous quote by Norton Juster: 'Expect everything so that nothing comes unexpected.' Leadership is about the same. Where would one find an example of this sort? Well, there are thousands of stories. History of 2019 onwards would also quote such examples, wherein leadership from all spheres would have been found to have exemplified the art of expecting everything and preparing for the unexpected. Around 17 June 2021, the medical science leadership projected a third wave in India with a huge magnitude and repercussions. The same day, markets were opened after around seven weeks for slightly a prolonged duration. The pictures of crowds without masks aggravated the projection of repercussions. Political leadership around the world has been acknowledging the virus waves. Europe met the third wave in June and the fourth wave also reached many places. Are these waves related to a compulsive response of the virus by mutating and spreading during the unlocks and people resorting to their routine with their imbibed mass behaviour gap and then succumbing and falling back to the locks? Is this that 'unexpected' to be 'expected' by the leadership? If it is, then preparing for the same should require the prolonged will of people to fight this war, accumulation of resources and, most of all, everyone doing whatever one should. How can people be led to that 'should'? Is there something which may be thought of as a precedence for the system at large? Are we missing the point that we are entrapped in our own compulsions? A dead organism which uses the human body to be alive, thrive and multiply has to be stopped. Strengthen the immune system of the body. Vaccinate the body. Isolate the infected. Once the immunity reduces, vaccination takes time and its effects will be there only for a certain period of time as they say. Isolation of infected can be done, but the virus spreads to others before revealing its presence in one. We can very well see that we do need a system where every participant knows about what is to be done and what should be done.

How to generate a self-regulated system? Do we have historical benchmarks and description? Is it Ram Rajya we are referring to? Thousands of papers have been written on the subject. There are books, documentaries, structured courses and thesis elaborating the elements of this system which has a guiding strength. The world requires anything and everything to learn from.

But first a few suggestions and a disclaimer.

Please don't take it as a religion-specific quote or term. The discussion here is not meant to bring up a religious discourse. Such discussions do invite varied reactions and responses. A spontaneous reaction to the reference of the relevance of this system which I have read and heard is how a scientific event like a pandemic can be met with a system like Ram Rajya? Here, it is important for the readers to understand that you may name it as any of the systems you remember but here the intent is to learn from everywhere.

There definitely are several other references, which might be quoted, but this book is about sharing an anguish about a pandemic which has affected all of us. I as an author understand 'Ram Rajya' as a system and do not intend to project it in comparison to other systems. Several universities, institutions, governments, organisations and nations which have been adapting and discussing it as an ideal social, political and economic system and a methodological framework have been acknowledging its relevance. It is the same Ram Rajya Mahatma Gandhi has mentioned which said that 'the ancient ideal of Ramarajya is undoubtedly one of true democracy in which the meanest citizen could be sure of swift justice without an elaborate and costly procedure' (For further details you may access to a search engine of your choice and several websites referring to the subject. For example: https://www.mkgandhi.org/momgandhi/chap67.htm).

Let's Talk a Little Bit More about the Enemy

An unseen, self-multiplying enemy, with a capability of developing several mutations as if a character who knows its capacities, understands the weaknesses of living beings, especially homosapiens, along with being an expert in catching the world unaware, which it has done with every wave. As if this virus has also been observing the socio-economic conditions and limitations of this globalised world and understands where to hit the hardest, how to spread, how to try to cause damage and probably understands the time humans might take to respond, fight back and weaken it.

What could have steered us? Who could have taken us out of this situation? Of course it is the frontline warriors, motivated and led by a committed leadership at all levels.

The enemy made us see and realise the worth of our leadership at both the micro and macro levels. A strong and motivated leadership came to the fore, committed to fight and lead us through, while building up a strategy, simultaneously fighting hard from the first day steering their teams and preparing for a tougher battle every day.

At the national level, the leadership came forward, addressed the people with strong hope, committing itself while motivating the nation for extending its commitment at al levels, as if challenging the virus to show its strength by making it realise that it won't be able to move forward at its own will.

Leadership Is Always Expected to Be Ideal

Leadership has a context of being related to vision and be human-centered. In today's scenario, we seem to have come far away from being human-centric and vision-related because we have started deciphering vision in terms of tangibility and the scales of development not revisiting the scales and measurement criteria but incrementally following those even at the cost of losing the context of distribution of the fruits of development at large. The means of development are being followed linearly following the changes we sought through advancement, turning it into an irreversible and non-deaccelerating process, which does not always carry along the participants who cannot run along or who get tired along the way. It sounds rhetorical but it is the leadership which decides on the change of course and change of perspective. It is the leadership which has to decide the precedence history would take.

India is fortunate to have leadership at all levels which has seen a vision of prosperity for all. The pandemic has brought the vision of our leaders to the fore once again. Leaders like Mahatma Gandhiji had wished for a self-reliant India, and this is also now the dream of the present leadership leading India towards Vocal for Local and Make in India. Any hesitation which was present in the adoption of this thought is pushed aside and now India is Vocal for Local. This banyan tree seemingly small at this stage is destined to grow in due course of time, wherein a decade from now the aspiring young generation would focus on contributing in this endeavour.

How to Look at Leadership?

Leadership is about going from subjectivity to objectivity and further to absolute. How does one move from being subjective to absolute? The answers are debatable. We all understand leadership is associated with ideals, beliefs and values. Though a simplistic answer may be that leaders emanate trust through their eyes, words and persona, and people follow them till their tangibility is realised. This belief in transition is what is leadership. We all have heard the stories of glorious battles fought by our soldiers under the command of strong commanders.

One must acknowledge COVID-19, which has now traversed into 2021, is definitely a learning phase in transition. It is continuously playing a puzzling game with this world wherein the latter has to ensure that the number of infected people has to be reduced, the number of fatalities has to be reduced to zero if possible, the economies must run, people must have the resources to live and a balance must be maintained alongwith a major obstacle that people might not be proactively cooperative in following the safety protocol. The most important part of the puzzle is that, though strong remedial measures and protocol including the most commendable vaccination drive is in place to help one and all, the virus has not revealed all its characteristics and the timing of reduction of its strength of multiplicity and effect.

This war as we all have seen has to be led to its culmination. Historians would definitely do justice in detailing the fact that it is the leadership at the macro and micro levels which kept on steering people and the situation and kept on fighting the enemy while trying to find out the key to its destruction, also documenting the fact that in future some other situation with a similar or different face might evolve. Though we wish and pray that the world becomes a better place and we live happily, the learning is that we can live in harmony with each other without greed and despair. Hope is the key and leadership holds it while unlocking our potential to live for each other.

How to Realise Values in Real Life

There are two ways, which I have found, and we all know that.

For realising values in day-to-day life, one has to discuss values through discussions and true stories.

Try to tell yourself that the values which you wish to nurture are not only to be discussed but are also to be transferred to the next generation.

It seems idealistic but the glory and preciousness of one's life for the reasons explicitly known to all of us especially proven and emphasised in the times of COVID-19 has compelled us many a time to adopt and strengthen our values and many a time to abandon those.

Leadership deciphers prosperity? Ram Rajya is one of those examples. Why? Because it specifically refers to follow '*Nij Nij Dharm*' – (one's own duties) although Dharma must be elaborated in a much larger context. But what is *Nij Dharm*? And who is going to tell us that?

I will come back to this in the end, as going along I remember one of the principals of one of the schools I attended who used to say that the face is the index of mind and smile is the index of heart. I never knew that after my education I would be a part of the business world for many years and then would come to education by becoming an academician at an institution like IIT Roorkee and would be reiterating those words before my students, which my sir used to say. I also remember the words of my teacher Shri Shanti Swaroop Vermaji who taught me mathematics when I was young. He always used to tell me 'if you have a question in your mind, pen in your hand and a blank paper in front of you, there is no way that you won't get an answer.' Believe me, many a time I have that kind of a situation. I'm the only one who has to take a call or decision and to bring up a solution to a huge practical problem given to me. My pen is before me, as is a blank paper, and I have to bring in solutions. Those solutions can be related to my day-to-day work, the subjects I teach, my administrative work, my consulting assignments or anything else. The submission here is that leaders say those words which enlighten you and lead you even if they are not there present physically? 'Leadership is a guiding force'. The force which generates a self-propelled system, where everyone knows his duty and lives for his responsibilities; there is not much space for one's own life. You would not spare a doctor who would not serve you in times of need, especially in case of situations like a pandemic. You would expect him to remember his 'Dharma'. This is true for everyone. Have you seen soldiers forgetting their duties? You would have to search for an answer. On 25 June, when we were finalising the draft, a discussion was going on about the days when all of it began. The three of us are academicians, who got engaged in our education-dissemination plan and contacting students through web and one of us is a senior editor of the government affairs with a television news channel who had to go out and bring the ground realities to the country. Should I be writing more about '*Nij Dharma*' or 'स्वधर्म'? This is where we search for a system to be developed. 'Ram Rajya'.

Let's refer to the quatrains below and I also present a gist according to my understanding for all the readers. (For translation please also refer to any website of your choice.)

रामराज्य

1. दैहिक दैविक भौतिक तापा। राम राज नहिं काहुहि ब्यापा॥
सब नर करहिं परस्पर प्रीती। चलहिं स्वधर्म निरत श्रुति नीती॥

In the whole of Sri Rama's dominions there was none who suffered from the affliction of any kind—whether of the body or proceeding from divine or supernatural agencies or that caused by another living being. All men loved one another: each followed one's prescribed duty, conformably to the precepts of the Vedas.

Kaand-Uttar Kaand
Chaupai 20, Line 1

2. अल्पमृत्यु नहिं कवनिउ पीरा। सब सुंदर सब बिरुज सरीरा॥
नहिं दरिद्र कोउ दुखी न दीना। नहिं कोउ अबुध न लच्छन हीना॥
सब निर्दंभ धर्मरत पुनी। नर अरु नारि चतुर सब गुनी॥
सब गुनग्य पंडित सब ग्यानी। सब कृतग्य नहिं कपट सयानी॥

There was no premature death nor suffering of any kind; everyone was comely and sound of body. No one was destitute, afflicted or miserable; no one was devoid of auspicious marks. All were unaffectedly good, pious and virtuous; all were clever and accomplished—both men and women. Everyone recognised the merits of others and was learned and wise; nay, everyone acknowledged the services and benefits received from others and there was no guileful prudence.

Kaand-Uttar Kaand
Chaupai 20, Line 3 and 4

3. फूलहिं फरहिं सदा तरु कानन। रहहिं एक सँग गज पंचानन॥
खग मृग सहज बयरु बिसराई। सबन्हि परस्पर प्रीति बढ़ाई॥
कूजहिं खग मृग नाना बृंदा। अभय चरहिं बन करहिं अनंदा॥
सीतल सुरभि पवन बह मंदा। गुंजत अलि लै चलि मकरंदा॥

Trees in the forest blossomed and bore fruit throughout the year; the elephant and the lion lived together as friends. Nay, birds and beasts of every description had forgotten their natural animosities and developed friendly relations with one another. Birds sang and beasts fearlessly moved about in the woods in distinct herds, making merry all the time. The air breathed cool, soft and fragrant; bees hummed even as they moved about laden with honey.

Kaand-Uttar Kaand
Chaupai 22, Line 1 and 2

(Goswami Tulsidasji. *Shri Ramcharitmanas*. Gorakhpur, UP: Gita Press, 2019.)

The quatrains above may be deciphered as this: none of the problems exist, and if arises it does not become prominent in Ram Rajya. Neither it is an idealistic situation nor hypothetical, not just because of the reason that it practically existed and that scriptures describe it at a great length but also because of the reason that a beautiful balance was created and nurtured by the leadership and maintained by people, therefore, avoiding any sorts of situations which may have created problems.

It simply means that people knew their duty and cared about what is to be followed and how humbly they could live while letting others live, which means if I cannot become the reason for the happiness for someone, I may also not become the reason for someone's problems and sorrows. Discipline, peace, integrity or values in totality bring in health, happiness, prosperity, harmony, environmental sustainability and all the other elements we have desired for, especially when we have witnessed problems beyond control or dire circumstances. Now please don't think that only science has to deal with environmental sustainability as we know science is not the answer to our greed.

Are you still wondering about what does COVID-19 have to do with an effective and efficient system? Or are we together on this point now?

Ram Rajya is historical and holds the key to a balance for prosperity. It is an expression of the result of leadership at the top-most level percolating down to the leadership at all functional levels and demonstrating a self-propelled system understanding the importance of integrity, commitment and will to face what may come.

Inculcating such a lesson and structuring a system for forthcoming generations will be a gift for them. I imagine a reader, years from now, who finds himself living with a great system with gratitude towards the predecessors while reading this text and feeling happy that we did think about our future and their present. JAI HIND.

4

Pandemic Narrative and the Mindset of Civil Society

RABINDRANATH BHATTACHARYYA

Once again there was a relief in the fourth week of June 2021. The curve of the second wave was flattening, although officially at the cost of more than 1.4 lakh lives.[1] But then the identification of the Delta+ strain in the blood samples from a number of states and more recently of the Omicron variant in some countries created a deep concern for the third wave and an imminent attack on children.

Amidst such apprehension, India has geared up with an aggressive vaccination drive. The shortage of vaccines on the one hand and a steep increase in awareness and desire for being vaccinated on the other have made the situation tough for both the central and state governments. Amongst a struggling vaccination drive, newer and newer horrible incidents came to the fore. The cost of funerals during the aggressive second wave led poor people to float the dead bodies of their loved ones in the Ganges. Seventy such bodies were recovered from the Ganges in Bihar and Uttar Pradesh[2] in the second week of May 2021. Hundreds of bodies were also buried along the banks of the river in Prayagraj[3] as it was found in the third week of May 2021. The oxygen crisis reached staggering proportions. In many hospitals, people died gasping for oxygen.[4] In the middle of this horrid and panic-stricken situation, the civil society expressed a resolute fight against the pandemic on the one hand and expressed a fatalistic approach towards corruption and immorality on the other.

Pandemics in History

This is not the first time that a pandemic has brought such a quandary in civil society. The first recorded pandemic of plague started in Athens in 430 BC, in the second year of the Peloponnesian War. Also, one hundred years back came the Spanish flu pandemic of 1918. Experts and scholars from various fields have been comparing the Spanish flu and COVID-19 with the help of existing literature, in terms of duration, number of fatalities, number of waves or the behaviour of civil society. Going by the experiences of all the three pandemics, we can observe that the community and voluntary organisations of society responded to pandemics in an unpredictable manner. The responses could vary from being helpful to being harsh to being agitated as resource crunch and administrative lacunae hit.

The great historian Thucydides, who himself was infected by the plague and evidenced the painful sufferings of other diseased persons of his society, gave a traumatic narration of the symptoms of and sufferings from the plague in his book *The Peloponnesian War*

Book II (Oxford World's Classic). He said the plague developed fast among the citizens of Athens. During the plague, Thucydides noticed some unexplained behaviour of nature too, as deaths rose. He said birds and animals, too, kept away from the dead bodies that were left unburied (Thucydides 2009, 98). Thucydides also gave a detailed count of the total number of deaths. 'It (the plague) killed no fewer than four thousand four hundred of the serving hoplites and, three hundred of the cavalry, and the number of deaths among the general populace is beyond computation.'[5] During the Peloponnesian War, the total population of Athens was over 300,000 (Hanson, 2005). Robert J. Littman estimated the count of death due to the plague in Athens to be 'perhaps as many as 75,000 to 100,000 people, 25% of the city's population died' (Littman 2009, 456). This was a huge number and the scale of the calamity rattled civil society in such a manner that the Athenians became demoralised. '(T)here was nothing that did more than the plague to demoralise the Athenians and damage their military strength'[6], Thucydides said.

The same was true about the community response during the Spanish flu. Historian Alfred Crosby, in his book *America's Forgotten Pandemic—The Influenza of 1918*, cited the official British history of the pandemic to say that the composite number of deaths in India in October 1918 had no 'parallel in the history of disease'(Crosby 2003, 207).[7] Crosby also cited Kingsley Davis, who viewed that only in the Indian subcontinent 20 million people died due to the pandemic (Davis 2003, 207). Crosby observed that the Spanish flu took more lives than any other disease in the world of a similar duration (Crosby 2003, 215). Authors such as Gina Kolata (2005, 5)[8] noted that these were very harrowing experiences of the pandemic that the people who had lived through it would not even want to talk about the experience.

In the wake of COVID's second wave, more than 3 crore people in India were infected up till the end of June 2021. Of them, officially more than 2.93 crore have recovered and around 3.97 lakh people died.[9] However, on 6 May 2021 Reuters reported, quoting an analysis of the Institute for Health Metrics and Evaluation (IHME) of the University of Washington, that the pandemic had caused nearly 6.9 million deaths in the world, which was more than double the official death number.[10] The *New York Times* reported on 25 May 2021 that in consultation with more than a dozen experts, an analysis of the number of COVID deaths in India till 24 May 2021 found that the number was 6 lakh.[11] The *Hindustan Times* on 13 June 2021 reported that the 'pandemic toll rises as states reconcile numbers'.[12] So, there remains a question about the real number of death as well as number of COVID-infected persons.

During the first wave, the Indian government took stringent measures and imposed a nationwide lockdown in four phases from 25 March 2020 to prevent the virus from spreading, to ramp up health infrastructure and to make people understand that they needed to take the issue a lot more seriously. But after the devastating second wave, the central government vested the responsibility of restricting citizens to the states. The vaccination programme, despite shortages in jabs and various changes in policy, continued. At first, the central government made vaccines available for all COVID frontline warriors like doctors, nurses, police personnel, etc. Then they were made available to all citizens above 60 years and over 55 years who suffered from co-morbidities (which was later on lowered to over 45 years irrespective of co-morbidities) free of cost at government institutions. On 23 April 2021, the central government declared that vaccines were available to everyone over the age of 18 years at any private vaccination centre for a cost.[13]

The Supreme Court then, in its 31 May 2021 order, contradicted the reasons of the central government on three issues of vaccination policy: decentralised procurement of vaccines, differential pricing and paid vaccination for citizens in the 18–44 age group under its 'Liberalised Vaccine Policy'.[14] Finally, the prime minister in his 7 June 2021 address to the nation declared vaccination for the 18–44 age group as free of cost, with the central government distributing vaccines to the states. However, throughout the period of the surge of second wave, there was a shortage of vaccine doses. The central government, citing the reason of efficacy of the vaccine, increased the gap between two Covishield doses to 12–16 weeks on 13 May 2021. The speed of inoculation varied from state to state, although sections of the public realised that the sooner everyone was immunised, the faster the economy would be back on track.

Pandemic and Its Grip on Social Lives

The term pandemic was first used by Gideon Harvey in 1666 in his book *Morbus Anglicus*. He wrote a chapter titled 'On the Original, Contagion, and Frequency of Consumptions',[15] making it coterminous with epidemic or endemic. The first serious attempt to define and clarify the term was possibly made by Dr Lawrence K. Altman, in his article 'Is This a Pandemic? Define "Pandemic"', published in the *New York Times* on 8 June 2009, as a response to the sudden outbreak and rapid global spread of a novel H1N1 influenza virus. Altman defined the pandemic as fundamentally a new agent that results from global transmission.

On 24 February 2010, WHO defined a pandemic as 'the worldwide spread of a new disease'.[16] Three other features should be added to these though, namely, high contagiousness, severity and minimal population immunity.[17] Going by these, COVID is certainly a pandemic.

Once a pandemic is declared, the state begins to control an individual's social life to a great extent. For instance, the mandate for wearing masks and limitations on visiting friends and family was issued. Mobile applications such as the Aarogya Setu app were used to track and trace COVID patients. Consequently, society responded to such state initiatives either in the form of appreciation and obedience or resistance and defiance, thereby responding to the etiological uncertainty of the contagion.

As analysts, if we go through at least some of these responses, we may identify some major features of a broader narrative—a narrative that tells us about the lessons that can be gleaned from the painful experiences of the pandemic and how it connects state–civil society relations in a pandemic situation.

Mask Mandate, Social Distancing and Stigma

In a pandemic, people's behaviour makes a lot of difference in controlling the spread of the virus and slip-ups can cost lives. For example, in India itself we saw people who were wearing masks in 2020 stopped doing so in the next year.

In October 1918, Dr William Hassler, chief of San Francisco's Board of Health, along with all the other board members advocated to the Board of Supervisors that wearing masks in any public place was compulsory for everyone in the city. Accordingly, a mask ordinance was passed in San Francisco that any person in any public place or in any place where two or more people were present or anybody involved with the sale, handling or delivery of foodstuff must wear masks 'consisting of four-ply materials known as butter-cloth or fine mesh gauze'.[18] However, even when the fatalities peaked during the Spanish flu, there were many people who resisted the mandatory wearing of masks in public places on the pretext that it was 'uncomfortable', 'inconvenient', 'fogged up one's spectacles', 'brought on attacks of neuralgia'[19] or that it was 'subversive of personal liberty and constitutional rights'.[20]

During the initial phase of the COVID crisis, there were no standard operating procedures (SOP) in place. The first guidelines on the pandemic came from the Ministry of Health and Family Welfare (MoHFW), Directorate General of Health Services in India, in the second week of March 2020. It said: 'Persons having no symptoms are not to use a mask.'[21]

However, on 4 June 2020, in a notification on the SOP on preventive measures to contain the spread of the virus in offices, the ministry said: 'Use of face covers/masks to be mandatory.'[22] This mandate has been reinforced by the order of the Ministry of Home Affairs, Government of India, dated 23 March 2021, which authorises states and union territories to impose fines in case of someone not wearing a mask in public and work spaces and spitting in public places [Order No. 40-3/2020-DM-I(A)]. The union and state governments began to spread awareness about the guidelines for wearing masks, cleaning hands with soap or sanitisers and the importance of keeping a six-feet distance between two people through various media, including a voice message for all telephone and mobile callers and through advertisements on TV and radio.

Starting from April 2020, many cities such as Kolkata, Delhi and Chennai imposed fines for not wearing masks in public places either under the Epidemic Diseases Act, 1897, or under the Indian Penal Code. Since July 2020, some states like Kerala have made it mandatory for people to wear masks or face covers in keeping with COVID guidelines. The Kerala Epidemic Disease Corona Virus Disease (COVID-19) Additional Regulations, 2020, notified that in all public places, work places and in all kinds of vehicles and transport every person must cover their mouth and nose with masks/face covers and in case of repeated violations, there will be a fine of ₹10,000.[23] In Jharkhand, the penalty for non-compliance was ₹1 lakh and a jail term up to two years.[24] In Gwalior, a novel type of penalty was introduced; people who did not wear masks or who did not follow COVID-19 protocols in public places were directed to work as volunteers in hospitals and police checkposts for three days.[25]

Unlike now, there were no mass media channels such as the radio, television or social media like Facebook or WhatsApp during the Spanish flu in 1918. So, mass awareness campaigns were run in newspapers or via notices in public places. In present times, despite the mass awareness campaigns on the importance of wearing masks, people in various parts of India have been seen defying the mask rule. As fear of contracting the virus started waning in the latter part of 2020, large sections of the population behaved irresponsibly and carelessly. They threw caution to the wind, especially during election campaigns in West Bengal, Assam, Kerala, Tamil Nadu and Puducherry, which led to the spread of the second wave.

People were seen resisting pandemic-related restrictions because of two reasons. One, there was a kind of complacency that the pandemic will not touch their lives. The other reason was that the restrictions would endanger their economic and institutional interests. Moreover, people were apprehensive about the social stigma attached to the pandemic and felt it could hamper their chances of getting work.

The catastrophic impact of the crisis has brought to the fore the ways by which society at large perceived the pandemic. During both waves, there was an element of social stigma attached to those infected with the virus along with disdain towards doctors attending to coronavirus-infected patients. During the first wave, doctors were either threatened by landlords to vacate their houses or harassed by patients' families. Such harsh behaviour demoralised the doctors. The situation went to such an extent throughout India that on the Writ Petition (Civil) [Diary No. 10852 of 2020],[26] the Supreme Court gave an order that necessary police security be extended to doctors and other medical staff treating COVID patients, and the state was directed to take necessary action against those persons who obstruct and commit any offence with respect to performance of duties of doctors, medical staff and other government officials deputed to contain the virus. This was just one of the many examples of how the pandemic created a lack of trust within the community, thereby triggering unpredictable responses from the society in general. At the same time during the tsunami of the second wave, many civil society networks sprang into action and provided oxygen and medicines and delivered food to patients. In West Bengal, Red Volunteers, Green Volunteers and various university students' bodies that networked for providing these services earned appreciation from the mass media. In some cases, like the Red Volunteers or Green Volunteers, these organisations are directly linked to the party; although there were other voluntary community-level organisations as well.

The stigma associated with the disease also increased caste violence in India. Social distancing was a traditional practice associated with casteism in India, in accordance with the Brahmanical concept, where the higher castes kept a social distance from the lower rungs of the caste hierarchy. During the pandemic, people from the lower castes, especially Dalits, faced a greater amount of social ostracism and atrocities. The use of the term 'social distancing' underpinned caste exclusion and caste violence during the pandemic, especially during the lockdown. There was a rise in incidents of violence against Dalits. The National Dalit Movement for Justice (NDMJ), a rights-based organisation for the Dalits, publicised the rising attacks on the community in April and May 2020, which was 72 per cent higher than such numbers in April and May 2019.[27] Dalits were shunned by the higher castes even from the same occupation. On 2 June 2020, the online edition of *US News* published an article by Sumit Ganguly with the headline 'India's Coronavirus Pandemic Shines a Light on the Curse of Caste.'

Two Very Different Worlds of Leisure

Thucydides observed that due to the plague there was 'increased lawlessness in the city'.[28] The people in Athens lifted their inhibitions from enjoying some pleasures during the plague that earlier occurred in a covert manner. Thucydides cited two reasons for that. Firstly, some people had become rich overnight after they amassed the property of prosperous family members who had died in the pandemic. These people began to behave recklessly, indulging in leisure activities believing 'that neither life nor wealth would last long.' The second reason was: 'no fear of god or human law was any constraint.'

Citing from Boccaccio's *The Decameron*, Gina Kolata spoke about two extremes during the Spanish flu. Gina spoke about one group of extremely scared citizens who locked themselves at home and could, therefore, remain untouched by the pandemic. These people even refrained from speaking to outsiders or receiving news of the dead. They would consume a modest amount of food and wine and would keep themselves entertained by listening to music, which is a matter of eudaimonic entertainment. On the other extreme were those who drank heavily and wouldn't let go of any opportunity to enjoy life to the hilt. This, of course, was a matter of hedonic pleasure.

During the two waves of the recent pandemic, the world of entertainment in India underwent unforeseen changes. Movie theatres were shut throughout the country since 25 March 2020. Live events such as musical programmes or plays, which were pivotal parts of our socio-cultural lives across states and languages, came to a complete halt. Tourism, too, came to a screeching stop.

Outside the containment zones, the Ministry of Home Affairs allowed movie theatres to run at 50 per cent capacity from 15 October 2020[29], under its guidelines for the fifth phase of the unlock. Since 1 February 2021, the government allowed 100 per cent occupancy in movie theatres. But in the wake of the second wave, most states declared strict restrictions, which included shutting down of all movie theatres. India's live events market, estimated to reach ₹12,200 crore by 2022 from the ₹8,300 crore in 2020,[30] suffered huge losses during this pandemic. Programme sponsors, too, were in a very tight spot due to lockdown-induced closures.

The Events and Entertainment Management Association (EEMA), as reported in *ET Brand Equity* (dated 21 April 2020), conducted a survey of 170 member companies affected by the first wave of the pandemic. One of the key findings of the report was that between March and July 2020 almost 52.91 per cent companies said 90 per cent of their businesses were cancelled. At the same time, big sports events were also halted. So, OTT platforms and home-based entertainment stepped in to fill that void. In urban areas, other than television, digital and online platforms became the channels for entertainment. In the initial week of the national lockdown, 'India's total TV consumption grew by 37 per cent to cross a record 1.21 trillion minutes'.[31] The same was reported by Shyamala Venkatachalam, who observed that such consumption of television programmes was neither witnessed nor imagined ever before.[32]

Any online medium of entertainment is inherently individualistic, whether it involves hedonic or eudaimonic entertainment motivations. The pandemic slowly but steadily created an entertainment culture of individualism among Western-educated, comparatively rich and urbane people, which would have a distinct motivating impact upon the culture enmasse. Rural India, however, still goes with traditional collectivistic culture that exists within ethnic identities as well as majority/minority identities. The complex social, religious and cultural practices of these identities coexist with low Human Development Index. In many cases, these cultural practices go against the ethical framework to fight a pandemic. The cross-societal differences in cultural dynamics have an impact on the responses to the pandemic, which is revealed through less awareness and less acceptance of social regulations in a collectivist culture. This becomes obvious especially in religious congregations like the Kumbh Mela. At the Kumbh Mela 2021 in Haridwar, there were provisions for three *shahisnans* held on 12, 14 and 27 April. Seventy lakh devotees participated. However, the Mela was scaled down midway due to fear of it becoming a super-spreader event.[33] Nevertheless, with state sanction for the congregation on the one hand and increase in television viewership on the other, the pandemic gradually facilitated a process of acculturation. This process reflected the values of the ruling elite for social life in general.

Shades of a Pandemic

Two important features were observed during the plague of Athens, one of which was strikingly common with the Spanish flu. First, the plague struck the residents of Athens in two waves. It came the first time in the summer of 430 BC and lasted for two years.[34] It made a second appearance in the winter of 427 BC. Thucydides observed that after the first wave that lasted two years, the plague never disappeared entirely, although it provided some remission. The next wave lasted for less than a year. So, the plague was there in totality for four-and-a-half years with some remission after the first wave. The second feature is that the plague never went beyond the Attica region in Greece between

430 BC and 427 BC. The original outbreak of the plague, though, was possibly in Ethiopia from where it spread to Egypt and Libya, and then it hit Athens. The plague of 430 BC spread over a few states of Africa and Europe, whereas the Spanish flu exploded in the four continents of Africa, Europe, America and Asia.

The Spanish flu, too, had two distinct waves, although Crosby spoke about a third wave as well that basically corresponded with the second one. In March 1918, the first wave started by infecting the 15th US Cavalry and then spread to Europe. In the initial stages, there were just 36 cases and six fatalities.[35] Then, it spread across borders to many cities. However, the virus mutated during the end of August 1918 and then spiralled with unparalleled severity 'in the same week in three port cities thousands of miles apart: Freetown, Sierra Leone; Brest, France; and Boston, Massachusetts'.[36] It stayed for about one year in two waves: March 1918 to March 1919.

The coronavirus spread across the globe in a span of just three months, after having originally exploded in China in December 2019, as today's world is a much more globalised one and there is frequent mobility across borders. However, the virulence of the second wave of the current pandemic in India was equivalent to the second wave of the Spanish flu. On 19 June 2021, The *Guardian*, quoting an anonymous scientific adviser, reported that in the UK there has been a surge of a 'third wave' while the vaccination programme intends to outpace the spread of the Delta variant of the virus.[37] In fact, on 4 June 2021, *Republic World* mentioned that Europe has been battered with the third wave of COVID.[38] It is this virulence of the disease that spread panic amongst people. In the case of COVID, advanced medical knowledge and the surveillance of contagion could also make people hyperaware of the pandemic threats they had been previously ignorant of. The extent of the panic in all these pandemics may be understood if we take up few cases.

Thucydides said once people realised that they had contracted the plague, they were shattered and very scared. So, they almost surrendered to the disease. Such kind of apprehensions often leads to panic and certain morbidity. During the current pandemic, news channels telecast various bits of bizarre news and this often pressed the panic button. Social media, although not always, created frenzy by spreading baseless rumours. While there is panic on the one hand, there is social stigma on the other. Thus, we find that be it the plague of Athens, the Spanish flu or COVID, people are so terror-stricken that they do not want to go near the infected person even when the patient is in dire need of help.

During COVID, patients were left to die on the streets, in ambulances or alone at home. As reported by the *Telegraph*'s online edition on 27 July 2020, a person named Madhab Narayan Dutta was admitted to a hospital in Bangaon on 25 July 2020 and was to be shifted to a COVID care unit in Kolkata. However, he was left to climb the waiting ambulance all by himself because even the PPE-wearing ambulance driver did not help him to get in. He was left alone with his wife by the side of ambulance. Unable to climb in without any help, he died there.

The *Indian Express* as well as *The Hindu* reported on 2 July 2020 that the body of a 71-year-old man, who had tested COVID-positive, had to be kept at home in a freezer for nearly 48 hours as the family members failed to secure help from government agencies and the police for the cremation.

On 20 April 2020, R.K. Radhakrishnan wrote in *Frontline* that in Chennai a mob attacked 'an ambulance that had arrived at a city burial ground with the body of Dr Simon Hercules, a neurosurgeon, who died of COVID-19 infection'. The Chennai police had to arrest 20 people in connection with that attack. The same report also mentioned that similar incidents occurred at Ambattur in Chennai, where a coronavirus infected doctor's body was prevented from being buried by a mob.

Of Last Rites and Dignity

According to COVID protocols, no one in any part of the world is permitted to take back the dead for the last rites. In every country, the last rites of COVID-infected dead bodies were performed by local authorities. On 15 March 2020, the directorate general of health services in India issued guidelines for management of bodies of patients who had died from suspected or confirmed COVID. The guidelines said the family will be allowed to see the body after maintaining social distancing protocol. However, there was panic in the community about the disease being highly infectious, and in the initial days there was an incident in West

Bengal where the locals did not allow the funeral rites of a COVID-infected person to go through.

On 24 March 2020, a 57-year-old man died in Kolkata of COVID. When his body was being brought for cremation, locals locked the gate of the crematorium. A huge police force ultimately dispersed the mob and the funeral took place around midnight. Sixteen people, including eight women, were arrested for rioting, unlawful assembly and for causing mischief.[39] Later, a legal case was instituted against the principal secretary of the Ministry of Health and Family Welfare, Government of West Bengal, and others at Calcutta High Court by Vineet Ruia, an active member of an NGO Bharat Bachao Sangathan. The court gave its verdict on 16 September 2020. The complainant said that the bodies of COVID patients were being disposed of in an unceremonious and undignified manner and close relatives were not allowed to pay their last respects. The complainant also raised the issue of lack of proper reporting of COVID-related deaths by the government and said there should be district-wise lists of patients. In its judgement, the Calcutta High Court said: 'We are of the firm view that the right of the family of a COVID-19 victim to perform the last rites before the cremation/burial of the deceased person is a right akin to Fundamental Right within the meaning of Article 21 of the Constitution of India.'

Despite the high court verdict, in the wake of the second wave, the dignity of COVID patients who had passed away was violated in a severe manner. Since the third week of April 2021, it was observed that in Delhi, Agra, Ahmedabad, Bengaluru, Ghaziabad, Lucknow and Varanasi—every place the second wave had aggressively hit—dead bodies had piled up at crematoriums and there was a 20-hour wait[40] at some places. Suddenly, it was felt that there was a massive shortage of crematoriums throughout the country. The heart-wrenching sight of dead bodies piled upon the pavement outside crematoriums was reported by the media.[41] At many places, many funeral pyres were lit together[42] and in others bodies were put together in a single funeral pyre.[43] In some cities, bodies were cremated on the pavement outside crematoriums.[44] Besides, on 19 May 2021, *BBC News* Delhi reported that 'Covid-19: India's holiest river is swollen with bodies'.[45] Dead patients belonging to the Christian and Muslim communities faced the same fate at cemeteries.

Election Frenzy amidst a Pandemic

Developing countries such as India, which got their independence after the Second World War, began to experience the problem of sustaining newly built institutions, of keeping alive high idealism and aspirations and of keeping them operative and efficient. Elections are the basic mechanism through which democratic institutions are sustained and remain operative. Consequent waves of the current pandemic posed a serious challenge to these democratic processes.

Parliament sessions were held for just 23 days in between 31 January and 1 March 2020 in the first phase and then from 14 September to 23 September 2020 without any break. Within these short sessions, many important bills like the three farm bills The Farmers (Empowerment and Protection) Agreement on Price

Assurance and Farm Services Bill, 2020, The Farmers' Produce Trade and Commerce (Promotion and Facilitation) Bill, 2020, and the Essential Commodities (Amendment) Bill, 2020, were passed hastily without much discussion. Those three farm laws were later withdrawn in Indian Parliament on 29 November, 2021. A comparison of the number of days of Parliament sessions in 2018 (the Lok Sabha elections took place in 2019) may highlight the paucity of Parliament sessions in 2020.

In 2018, the budget session continued from 29 January 2018 to 6 April 2018, monsoon session from 18 July 2018 to 10 August 2018 and the winter session from 11 December 2018 to 8 January 2019.[46] In 2021, the budget session started on 29 January 2021 and Parliament was adjourned on 25 March sine die due to the advent of the second wave of COVID. Within this period, 20 Bills (17 in Lok Sabha and 3 in Rajya Sabha) were passed.[47] During the pandemic in 2020, Bihar was the first state where elections were held—between 28 October and 7 November. At the same time, the US, too, had its presidential elections on 3 November 2020.

Then the elections in West Bengal, Assam, Kerala, Tamil Nadu and Puducherry were held from 27 March 2021 to 29 April 2021. West Bengal had eight phases of polls, which created a debate about the role of the Election Commission of India (ECI) in conducting elections during the second wave. Besides, in Maharashtra and Uttar Pradesh, Gram Panchayat elections were also organised in 2021. Huge election rallies, organised by all parties in each of these states, violated all pandemic norms and the ECI sat as a mute spectator. The deaths of 135 teachers, *shikshamitras* and investigators due to COVID after participating in poll duties led the Allahabad High Court to issue a notice to the state election commission as to why the poll officials responsible for COVID protocol violations should not be prosecuted.[48] Aspirations and demands addressed during election campaigning reflected pandemic issues that people faced. The demand for jobs from migrants who came back home during the lockdown became a major issue in the Bihar elections. Besides, the Bharatiya Janata Party (BJP) had promised free vaccines for all citizens in the Bihar election campaign and later in West Bengal, which brought sharp criticism from opposition parties.[49] Responding to a Right to Information petition, the ECI said on 31 October 2020 that such poll promises did not violate the model code of conduct. However, there was plenty of video evidence that showed how mass gatherings at election rallies violated the guidelines related to social distancing and mask wearing.

The mask mandate was a bone of contention of the US presidential elections. So much so that Republican presidential candidate Donald Trump mocked his opponent Joe Biden for wearing a mask. Despite the recommendations of the Centres for Disease Control and Prevention (CDC), the American society was divided. It seemed like wearing masks hurt the pride of the Americans.

Where Is the Qualitative Value?

We are living in a consumer-oriented utilitarian society. The criterion for the collective good is calculated here in terms of happiness for the greatest number in society. While that has a number of quantifiable dimensions, including an electoral dimension, it is very difficult to put some extraneous qualitative values such as human rights or equity that can override the utilitarian nature of individuals in our society. The responses to the pandemic are illustrative of that.

References

'Covid-19 Safety Guidelines Mandatory for a Year in Kerala; Rs10K Fine for Not Wearing Masks', *Hindustan Times*, 6 July 2020, https://www.hindustantimes.com/india-news/kerala-makes-following-covid-19-guidelines-mandatory-for-a-year/story-JdoqeqO7KsargqPeUKPvTO.html.

Express Web Desk. 2020. 'Jharkhand's "No Mask" Penalty – Up to ₹1 Lakh; Here's How Other States are Dealing with Covid Rule Violators', *Indian Express*, 23 July, https://indianexpress.com/article/india/jharkhands-no-mask-penalty-up-to-rs-1-lakh-heres-how-other-states-are-dealing-with-covid-rule-violators-6520089/.

Hanson, Victor. 2005. 'A War Like No Other', *The New York Times*, 23 October, https://www.nytimes.com/2005/10/23/books/chapters/a-war-like-no-other.html#:~:text=The%20Peloponnesian%20War%20pitted%20against,and%20plenty%20of%20coined%20money.

Javeri, Lakshmi Govindrajan. 2020. 'Reeling under COVID-19 Impact, India's Live Events Giants Mull Future Approach for Audience Changed by Pandemic', *First Post*, 25 June, https://www.firstpost.com/entertainment/reeling-under-covid-19-impact-indias-live-events-giants-mull-future-approach-for-audience-changed-by-pandemic-8437481.html.

Littman, J. Robert. 2009. 'The Plague of Athens: Epidemiology and Paleopathology.' *Mount Sinai Journal of Medicine, Wiley InterScience*, 76 (5): 456–467.

Mlambo-Ngcuka, Phumzile. 2020. 'Violence Against Women and Girls: The Shadow Pandemic', UN Women, 6 April, https://www.unwomen.org/en/news/stories/2020/4/statement-ed-phumzile-violence-against-women-during-pandemic.

Morens, David M., Gregory K. Folkers and Anthony S. Fauci. 2009. 'What Is a Pandemic?' *The Journal of Infectious Diseases, Oxford Academic*, 1 October, 200 (7): 1018–1021.

PTI. 2020. 'Not Wearing Masks in Gwalior? You'll End Up Volunteering at Hospital', *New Indian Express*, 6 July, https://www.newindianexpress.com/nation/2020/jul/06/not-wearing-masks-in-gwalior-youll-end-up-volunteering-at-hospital-2166103.html

5

COVID-19 and the Challenge of Crisis Communication

HIMANSHU SHEKHAR MISHRA

18 March 2020

It was a normal working day in the Parliament for a news reporter. I still vividly remember the date: 18 March 2020, to be precise. As COVID-19 positive cases were rising gradually in the country, we could strongly sense the growing uncertainty around us as a climate of fear and rumour-mongering had begun to spread panic.

While I was reporting on the parliamentary proceedings, I got a call from home around 5:00 P.M. My wife was agitated as she apprised me that panic buying had started in our neighbourhood in Ghaziabad. She told me there were widespread rumours about an impending nationwide lockdown and residents in our housing society were getting jittery and worried that the Ghaziabad administration was planning to close all shops and malls for an indefinite period. It was a distress call to alert me that people in our locality had started buying huge quantums of food items and stocks were fast disappearing from ration shops and grocery stores near our home. By the time I finished my work in Parliament and rushed back home, it was too late to buy food items my family desperately wanted to stock in this hour of growing uncertainty. I was shocked to see a huge queue outside a local grocery store near my home in Vasundhara, Ghaziabad, at around 7:00 P.M. After nearly 40 restless minutes in the queue, when I finally managed to enter the grocery store, most of the shelves were already empty. It seemed that a rowdy crowd had just ravaged the store and looted most of the food items. The store manager told me people were indulging in panic buying and they had bought huge stocks of food items.

By the time I reached home, news channels were flashing reports of panic buying in different parts of the National Capital Region (NCR) as well. Within 24 hours, the situation became so worrisome across many cities that the prime minister had to come forward to caution people not to indulge in panic buying. In his widely televised address to the nation on 19 March 2020, the first since the COVID-19 outbreak in India, the prime minister tried to assuage concerns of common citizens. He assured them that the government had initiated all necessary steps to ensure adequate supply of essential items such as milk, groceries and medicines and appealed to them to not hoard essential items.[1] However, the growing fear and uncertainty among the masses showed that the crisis communication protocol initiated by the central and state governments was not producing the desired results. In this climate of fear, people showed scant regard to the threat of contracting the virus by stepping into crowded grocery shops, especially at a time when COVID-19 positive cases were rapidly rising in the country. They paid no heed to the words of assurance from government agencies and local administration that shops selling essential commodities would be allowed to open everyday for a limited period. Soon, the irrational stocking of food materials and panic buying had created a new crisis —a demand and supply mismatch in the market, leading to shortage of food supplies and commodities in grocery stores and ration shops.

Spectre of an 'Unpredictable' Coronavirus

The COVID-19 crisis exposed India's lack of preparedness to combat a pandemic. In the first few weeks, the central and state governments struggled to formulate a cohesive strategy to combat the worst public health disaster in India's post-independence history. The challenge was compounded by an urgent need to sensitise more than a billion people in a short span of time to the threat an 'unpredictable' coronavirus posed to their lives. It was a gargantuan task to disseminate information about the symptoms, safety and social distancing protocol to millions of homes in urban and rural areas.

In the initial weeks, the common people had very limited understanding of the preventive steps required to protect themselves and their families from the coronavirus. The absence of a national crisis communication protocol to specifically deal with a COVID-19-like pandemic aggravated the crisis that had gripped the nation. In the absence of a national action plan to fight such a deadly pandemic, the government had to struggle to formulate an institutional response mechanism to contain the spread of the coronavirus. The prices of hand sanitisers and masks began to skyrocket as people scrambled to medical shops. The sudden surge in the demand led to complaints that some companies were indulging in profiteering by artificially creating shortage in the market. A medical shop owner in Delhi's popular Bengali Market, K.K. Goyal told me on 3 March 2020 that customers were indulging in panic buying of sanitisers even though there was sufficient stock available in his shop.[2]

This forced the government to step in and cap the price of hand sanitisers and masks. The late food and consumer affairs minister Ram Vilas Paswan tweeted that the retail price of a 200-ml bottle of hand sanitiser cannot be fixed above ₹100 per bottle and no shopkeeper could sell masks for more than ₹10 per piece till 30 June 2021[3].

Prime Minister Shri Narendra Modi himself took the lead to fill the gaps that existed by opening a direct line of communication with the citizens. In his first address to the nation during the coronavirus outbreak on 19 March 2020, the prime minister announced the imposition of a 14-hour *janta* curfew (people's curfew) on 22 March 2020, between 7:00 A.M. and 9:00 P.M.[4] warning the countrymen that the COVID-19 crisis had affected more countries than both the First and Second World Wars. The prime minister urged people to stay away from crowds and gatherings and avoid leaving their homes. He said:

> Yes, I acknowledge that many difficulties arise in such times, and there is an environment of apprehension and rumours. Many a times, our expectations as

> citizens are also not fulfilled. However, this crisis is so grave, that all fellow citizens must face these challenges with firm resolve and determination, amidst all these difficulties.[5]

He followed it with a detailed interaction with the heads of electronic media institutions through video conference on 23 March 2020. It was held just a day ahead of the imposition of a three-week-long nationwide lockdown.

According to a note issued by the PMO, Shri Modi told the heads of electronic media institutions that COVID-19 was a 'lifetime challenge' and urged them to communicate 'swiftly' and 'professionally' the decisions taken by the government through their news channels in an easy language. He called for dissemination of 'positive' communication to 'counter' the pessimism and panic among the people.[6]

It was a precursor to the imposition of a draconian lockdown protocol in the entire country. The prime minister appeared again on national television on 24 March 2020 to announce a three-week complete lockdown.[7] By this time, the fear of an 'unpredictable' virus had gripped the country. In this moment of uncertainty, incidents of panic buying continued in different parts of the country despite specific assurances from the prime minister that the centre and the states would ensure availability of essential commodities.[8]

Crisis Communication Protocol on COVID-19

The government initiated extensive public communication processes on national media platforms to address the fundamental concerns and fear every Indian had: What would happen if a person got infected with COVID-19? Through mass media campaigns, the government agencies publicised the requisite standard protocols. These related to the responsibilities of citizens to follow quarantine and self-isolation guidelines. A list of hospitals was identified to treat COVID-19 cases and quarantine centres were set up for affected people. Posters and billboards were put up to educate common citizens about the precautionary measures such as physical distancing, wearing a mask at all times in public spaces, keeping their homes ventilated, avoiding moving in crowds and cleaning hands at frequent intervals.

In an unprecedented move, to fill the gaps in crisis communication, Shri Modi addressed the nation five times just in a span of seven weeks, between 19 March 2020 and 12 May 2020. In this period, one of the most stringent lockdown guidelines were first imposed and a process of easing restrictions were also gradually initiated. This was the period when large parts of India remained virtually under siege.

There was a continuous rise in the number of coronavirus cases in India during this period. The union health ministry data showed the number of cases stood at 173 when Shri Modi first addressed the nation on 19 March 2020. On the day of the *janata* curfew, which was just three days later on 22 March, the number had climbed to 324 cases. On 24 March, it further rose to 467 confirmed COVID-19 cases. By the time the prime minister addressed the nation for the fifth time on 12 May 2020, there were 70,756 cases in the country. The frequency of the prime minister's address then began to decline. His sixth address to the nation happened more than six weeks later, on 30 June 2020, when the number of confirmed cases had risen to 566,841 in the country.

As the number of confirmed cases continued to rise at an alarming rate, the prime minister did not address the nation for more than three-and-a-half-months, 112 days to be precise. His seventh address to the nation took place on 20 October 2020, when India had recorded 47,000 new COVID-19 cases in a day, the lowest rise in a span of 24 hours since July 2020. The total number of infected people in the country on that day was 75,97,063, the second highest in the world after the United States.

In his series of widely televised addresses to the nation, the prime minister outlined the rationale behind the imposition of a nationwide lockdown and outlined the challenges India was facing in combating the COVID pandemic. Through interviews and media briefings, union ministers and senior officials, too, opened communication channels to disseminate important information to the citizens as the uncertainty grew and the number of coronavirus-infected patients continued to rise.

But these advisories and words of assurance by authorities could not assuage the concerns of many people. As government imposed restrictions on economic activities and industries, factories were closed in different parts of the country and millions of poor migrant workers and underprivileged people scrambled to stock whatever little food items they could buy to survive the lockdown.

Media networks soon started broadcasting horrifying images of poor migrant workers forced to undertake a treacherous journey back home with their families. With no public transport service in operation, millions of workers had no option but to walk on foot for hundreds of miles. India witnessed an unprecedented reverse migration, which was largely an outcome of the larger economic crisis in India in the aftermath of a stringent national lockdown. It became the defining image of the COVID crisis in India in the Indian and global media.[9]

First COVID-19 Case in India

The challenge COVID-19 pandemic posed for India was gargantuan in scale. It was a herculean task for the central and state governments to deal with the devastating impact of the pandemic on common people. Importantly, the official machinery had started work on a roadmap to combat it at least two months before the virus actually hit India. In the initial days of the coronavirus outbreak in China, India had taken the threat posed by the deadly pandemic seriously. Available official documents show that the government had started preparing for all eventualities much before the first corona virus case was confirmed in India.

Exactly five days before the first COVID-19 case was reported on 30 January 2020, I had reported on an important high-level meeting called by the prime minister's Principal Secretary P.K. Mishra to review India's preparedness to deal with any eventuality.

A media note issued by the PMO said senior officials of the Ministry of Health and Family Welfare had briefed the principal secretary to the prime minister on the state of hospital and laboratory preparedness, measures initiated to strengthen the capacity building of rapid response teams and the extensive surveillance activities being initiated on 25 January 2020. By then, around 20,000 passengers arriving by 115 flights at seven international airports had been screened.[10]

Though the national media discourse was dominated at that time by a high-pitch election campaign to elect a new assembly in Delhi and the Union Budget for 2020, which was to be presented on 1 February, in the last week of January 2021, I shot a series of ground reports on the impact of the economic slowdown and the expectations of different sectors from the finance minister who was giving final touches to her budgetary proposals. In fact, a day before the first case of COVID-19 was reported in Kerala, I covered an important election rally in outer Delhi (Amit Shah's rally on 29 January 2020).[11] The Delhi assembly election campaign was in full swing and the primary focus of the national media was on the high-pitch election campaign.

Amidst the din of the Delhi assembly elections, the first confirmed case of COVID-19 virus was reported from Kerala. Union health ministry issued an unusually short three-line press note, which said that an Indian student studying in Wuhan University, China, had tested positive for the novel coronavirus infection in a Kerala hospital.[12]

The cabinet secretary chaired a high-level meeting on the same day. It was decided that all passengers who had returned from China after 15 January 2020 would have to undergo a mandatory COVID-19 test. The GoI also issued orders to send all passengers who had arrived from China to home isolation. The government also urged Indian citizens to avoid a visit to China.[13]

As India woke up to the rising threat of the virus, the second confirmed case was reported from Kerala again. The health ministry note said the patient had a travel history from China.[14] Within 24 hours, the third case of coronavirus was reported. The case history was the same. The patient had a travel history from Wuhan in China.[15] In less than 100 hours, India had reported three confirmed cases of coronavirus.

The prime minister immediately stepped in and directed the constitution of a Group of Ministers (GoM) headed by the Union Health Minister Harsh Vardhan, with a mandate to continuously assess and strengthen India's readiness to combat the threat posed by the coronavirus.[16] In view of the growing urgency, the GoM met the same day. It reviewed the screening protocol for passengers arriving from China, the global hotbed of COVID at that time. It decided to temporarily suspend both the e-visa facility for Chinese passport holders and the facility for submitting applications online for the physical visa from China.[17]

First COVID-19 Debate in Parliament

As anger rose and the opposition parties began to raise questions on the government's strategy to combat the COVID-19 crisis, the issue came up for discussion in the Lok Sabha, the lower house of the Indian Parliament. The Health Minister Dr Harshvardhan briefed Members of Parliament (MPs) on the state of the pandemic in the country. He outlined the government's risk communication strategy, which involved distribution and dissemination of public communication material in regional languages.[18]

As the debate on the pandemic opened up, the union health minister faced difficult and complex questions from MPs from across the political spectrum. Nationalist Congress Party MP from Baramati in Maharashtra Supriya Sule categorically said that the MPs too were confused about the nature of the pandemic outbreak. She questioned the government's media strategy to share information on the 'unpredictable' virus with the nation. Ms Sule asked the health minister in the Lok Sabha:

> Could you do a daily briefing to the media so that there is only one story that goes out? In every channel some doctor is saying something. We do not know whom to believe and whom not to believe. So, could you take one guideline and speak regularly so that we all can speak in one voice and follow what the government gives us.[19]

Ms Sule's statement was reflective of the growing uncertainty about the 'invisible' virus which had begun to create panic in the country. Opposition MPs also raised questions about the loopholes in the government's strategy to control the spread of the virus. K. Kanimozhi, the DMK MP from Tamil Nadu, raised serious questions about the weak thermal scanning procedures followed by government agencies at international airports. Citing her personal experience, she argued in the Lok Sabha:

> I think thermal screening is not available at most of the airports. It is not there at all. I have gone myself to the airport to receive people who came from abroad. Thermal screening was not done there. I think that has to be done. The swab test is also not being conducted. Rather than having a thermal screening, they are asking the people who are coming back from foreign countries to reveal where all they have travelled on their own. I think that will not be sufficient. I also think that masks are not available.[20]

A week after the parliament debated the pandemic, the GoI decided on 12 March 2020 to suspend all visas (except diplomatic, official, UN/international organisations, employment, project visas) till 15 April 2020.

Union Civil Aviation Minister Hardeep Puri told me in Parliament: 'We have taken decisions that were necessary to take under the given circumstances. At our land borders, sea ports, airports—all places through which international passengers come inside India—we have initiated steps. Our systems are functioning well. We need to keep them under constant monitoring. We have decided to suspend all non-essential travel-related visas.'[21]

The Indian Railways followed suit within days. The then railway board chairman, V.K. Yadav, told me in an interview on 19 March 2020, after briefing a Parliamentary committee that people should avoid all non-essential railway travel for a few days. He said that if it was very essential to travel, they must ensure that they do not travel in groups and avoid all contact with fellow travellers during the train journeys.[22]

Rise in Television News Viewership

The first day of the lockdown on 25 March 2020 was an exceptional day at work. The streets of Ghaziabad were completely deserted. All shops were closed; all types of public transport services were banned. As I drove out of my housing society to take stock of the situation in my neighbourhood in Vasundhara, the fear was palpable everywhere. The coronavirus was an unknown, unpredictable enemy. A few vehicles of Uttar Pradesh policemen were patrolling the streets, strictly enforcing the lockdown guidelines. It seemed India was at war with itself. Newspaper vendors were told to stay away from apartment complexes. Indians had access to very few credible primary sources of information such as television news channels and radio networks.

As more than a billion Indians were forced to stay indoors for days on end, they frequently tuned in to television news for updates on the pandemic and to get a sense of how fellow Indians were coping with one of the most stringent lockdowns in history. The Broadcast Audience Research Council (BARC) and a media research firm Nielsen found in a joint study that news consumption on television news platforms spurted by 251 per cent in Delhi and 177 per cent in Mumbai in the fifth week of the lockdown. The BARC-Nielsen report also showed that TV viewership rose by one hour and twenty-six minutes in Delhi and one hour and forty-two minutes in Mumbai.[23]

Challenges of Reporting on COVID-19

The rise in television news viewership during the lockdown brought public glare on media coverage of the COVID-19 crisis. As demand for television news rose, reporters and camerapersons braved all odds to move out in the field to extensively document and report on the crisis perpetrated by the pandemic. Television journalists had to reformat their technical gadgets and accessories. We began to use long boom microphones to keep ourselves at a safer distance from those we were speaking with or interviewing. However, despite a stringent safety protocol to keep themselves safe while interacting with the subjects of their stories, many journalists got infected with COVID. In one such instance, 53 journalists in Mumbai tested positive in a special medical camp set up by the Brihanmumbai Municipal Corporation (BMC) in which a total of 171 mediapersons had given their samples.[24]

With production and shooting of films, television serials and national and international sporting events completely banned, the TV news channels were producing fresh content every hour, broadcasting images of how India was fighting the war against the pandemic.

Working in a climate of fear involved managing a lot of risks. Television news journalists had to reformat their workplace and reform their methodology of gathering news to keep both the manpower and workspace safe. They reformatted their equipment, especially boom mikes by increasing their length to ensure that they kept the subjects of news at a safer distance from themselves. As part of COVID-19 safety protocol, the entry of reporters into a newsroom was stopped and a large part of the staff was told to work from home. Many news organisations provided makeshift studio infrastructure at the homes of news anchors and reporters to minimise their exposure to the virus. The advent of mobile journalism facilitated the flow of information even from inside a containment zone. It helped in curtailing the hazards of news gathering during the worst public health disaster in India's history.

Covering a pandemic is potentially very hazardous. I devised my own safety protocol, based on a personal risk assessment plan that focused on reducing the exposure to unknown people, maintaining a safe distance while talking to people, using masks, sanitisers and all other necessary protective medical gear at frequent intervals. I also ensured that I travelled mostly in my personal vehicle or a thoroughly sanitised office vehicle. But despite these protective measures, a large number of mediapersons, especially reporters, camerapersons and on-field broadcast engineers, contracted the virus. The newsgathering processes were affected across many TV news channels. According to a study conducted by the Network of Women in Media, 165 Journalists had lost their lives to COVID-19 till 1 May 2021, with 60 deaths recorded in April alone during the deadly second corona virus wave (an average of two deaths every day).[25]

As media organisations grappled with the challenge to keep their reporting and editorial teams and production staff safe and continue with a seamless flow of news, they also had to contend with complex moral and ethical questions while broadcasting news. News channels had to formulate their editorial policies on what to report and what not to report. The first question we had to grapple with was how to protect the identity of COVID patients so as to save them from any kind of social ostracisation while highlighting their plights. Media institutions had to reformulate the conventional principles of news coverage and newsgathering processes. The identity of corona virus positive patients undergoing treatment was not revealed on TV channels.

Soon, the government initiated a process of frequent media briefings by the health ministry and the Indian Council of Medical Research (ICMR). This arrangement continued for a few weeks. However, as the cases continued to rise unabated, the frequency of these media briefings began to decline and the absence of ICMR's experts became a subject of media debate.[26] In fact, the announcement of extension of lockdown restrictions was made through written press releases by the home ministry as the COVID crisis deepened. The government became more defensive and briefings began to be held only intermittently at infrequent intervals.[27] There were incidents of journalists being targeted for covering developments related with COVID-19 crisis. In one such instance, on 10 July 2020, the Press Council of India (PCI) sought comments from the Uttar Pradesh government. The official press release said:

> The Press Council of India takes suo-motu cognisance regarding alleged targeting of journalists during the COVID-19 lockdown period in the state of Uttar Pradesh. In one incident an FIR has been lodged against four journalists in Gopiganj police station at Bhadohi district of Uttar Pradesh and in a separate incident a notice has been issued to Mr Vijay Vineet, reporter and Mr Subhash Rai, editor-in chief of *Jansandesh Times* for reporting on issues that concerns the plight of people during the lockdown period. Since the matters concern free functioning of the press the Hon'ble Chairman, Press Council of India has viewed the matters with concern and called for comments from the state government of Uttar Pradesh.[28]

Media coverage of the COVID-19 pandemic has been intensely debated at both national and international levels. There have been controversies too, especially with regard to the nature of coverage of Tablighi Jamaat Markaz (meeting), held in Nizamuddin in the national capital amid the pandemic, in sections of the electronic media. After a large number of coronavirus positive cases were reported among the stranded attendees at Nizamuddin, who had assembled from many countries to attend the Jamaat activities, the Tablighi Jamaat was vehemently criticised and allegations were levelled against it for violating lockdown guidelines.[29] A controversy arose over questions raised in some news channels about an alleged intent to 'vilify' and 'demonise' a religious community.

The Jamait Ulema-i-Hind filed a petition in the Supreme Court against the attempt in sections of the electronic media to blame an entire religious community for the spike in the infections and for deliberately targeting them.[30] In fact, at one stage during the hearing on 17 November 2020, the three-judge Supreme Court bench told Solicitor General Tushar Mehta: 'We want to know as to what is the mechanism to deal with these contents on television. If there is no regulatory mechanism then you create one.'[31]

India Begins to 'Unlock'

As the situation began to stabilise and the government became more confident in handling the COVID situation, a process to 'unlock' economic activities was initiated. The government began to ease lockdown restrictions in a graded way. Industries slowly restarted their operations. As industry and factory owners tried to restart production work, it soon became clear that the Indian economy had suffered an unprecedented contraction during the nationwide stringent lockdown.

I shot my first ground report in a small manufacturing unit of Toshi Automatic Systems Pvt. Ltd situated in Bulandshahar Road Industrial Area in Ghaziabad. Sanjeev Sachdev, the managing director of Toshi Automatic Systems which produces high-end automated products for industrial and commercial clients, told me that he was facing the worst financial crisis of his 34-year career. Facing a shortage of capital and supply- line bottlenecks, Sanjeev Sachdev admitted that he had managed to resume only 20 per cent of his business operations by the end of May 2020.[32] Shops of primary materials were still closed in many parts of the country, and he was struggling to restart production of high-tech automated systems. He said he was working hard to sustain his business through this unprecedented crisis. Overall, 30 to 40 per cent of the total 470 industrial units in Bulandshahar Road Industrial Area were still closed in May 2020.[33]

I met a large number of workers in Bulandshahar Road Industrial Area who were struggling to find work. Some who were lucky to find a job told me their daily income had fallen from an average of ₹400 to ₹500 per day in pre-COVID times to just ₹100 a day. On the same day, a national survey of micro, small and medium enterprises (MSME) units by the Federation of Indian Micro, Small & Medium Enterprises and SKOCH Group revealed that around 62 per cent of around 6.3 crore MSME units in the country had laid off workers, 30 per cent MSMEs were planning to cut 30 per cent of their staff and 26 per cent MSME units were planning to cut one-fourth of their staff while 78 per cent had decided to reduce salaries of workers.[34]

In an interview, the secretary general of the Ministry of Micro, Small and Medium Enterprises Anil Bhardwaj told me, 'Sixty-two per cent of the MSMEs who participated in the survey did not show confidence in the financial relief package announced by the union finance minister.'[35] But the situation gradually improved and the economy seemed to be coming back on rails as months progressed and more and more industrial centres and markets were opened over the next few months. By December 2020, the economy seemed to be recovering.

India Breathes Easy as COVID Numbers Fall

After battling uncertainty for almost 11 months, news reporters had begun to finally breathe easy when the number of new COVID-19 cases began to fall in January 2021. At one time, the number of daily new cases recorded nationwide reached as low as 9,102 on 26 January 2021, the lowest in eight months.[36] It raised hopes that India was moving closer to finally winning the war against the pandemic after battling it since 30 January 2020, when the first case was reported in Kerala of a medical student who had returned from Wuhan, China. As the new cases remained at a low trajectory, I chose to take a break from work after relentlessly reporting on the COVID-19 crisis for almost a year and decided to visit my hometown Bokaro Steel City in the state of Jharkhand, which had become 'largely' a COVID-free city. The process of 'unlocking' India was also gradually moving forward.

The family holiday in Bokaro was a revelation, as a majority of people had stopped using masks in the Steel City. It seemed like a return to the pre-COVID way of life. But it did not last long. As I began to pack up after almost two weeks to return to Delhi on 2 March 2021, a close school-friend Sanjay Kumar, who ran a diagnostic lab in the city, told me that two samples had turned positive within 24 hours. This was the first indication that COVID had begun to rear its head again in Bokaro. As I left Bokaro, a similar rise in new cases was being reported in several smaller towns and cities across the country, and some state governments had begun to reimpose travel restrictions.

Overcrowded Crematoriums, Mass Funerals Haunt the World

Within a month, it became clear that the spectre of COVID had returned to haunt India again. As the number of cases rose alarmingly, the national discourse began to change with the worst-affected states Maharashtra and Chattisgarh deciding to impose stringent lockdowns to contain the disturbing rise in COVID-19 infections. Within days, as the national capital Delhi reported an alarming rise in coronavirus infections, the Delhi government too was forced to impose a night curfew from 8 April 2021. The second coronavirus wave was far more lethal and destructive than the first wave; it was to change India forever. The state-wise lockdowns and restrictions failed to arrest the unprecedented rise in new COVID-19 infection cases. On 6 May 2021, the number of new cases reached a staggering 4,14,182, the highest recorded anywhere in the world since the COVID pandemic struck the world in late 2019.[37]

As bodies of COVID victims piled up outside crematoriums, the local administration in many cities had to make emergency arrangements to dispose them of as per official COVID protocol. Many cities reported a huge backlog, as crematoriums ran out of space to complete the funerals with due COVID protocol. The unprecedented images of crowded crematoriums piled up with dead bodies and scores of burning pyres published in the media became the image of this national crisis in leading international news media networks across the world. In some cities, when mortuaries could not dispose of the dead with COVID protocol in stipulated time, several makeshift mortuaries had to be constructed overnight to deal with large number of deaths. The absence of a well-defined funeral assistance protocol complicated the unprecedented humanitarian crisis. Poor families faced an acute crisis, as they struggled to arrange the funds needed to bid a final farewell to their loved ones. This was in sharp contrast to the funeral assistance programme initiated by the United States' nodal disaster management agency—the Federal Emergency Management Agency (FEMA)—on its integrated web portal. FEMA had actively provided state-specific funeral assistance information to families of COVID victims along with financial assistance to needy families[38].

India Fights for Oxygen

The failure of hospitals and healthcare systems in many cities to provide basic facilities like medical oxygen and critical medicines to the growing number of COVID patients led to a virtual collapse of the healthcare system as India battled to save lives during the peak of the second wave of the COVID-19 pandemic. 2 May 2021 marked an exceptional day at work of my two-decade long news-reporting career. I was positioned at the BJP headquarters on the day votes were being counted for five state assembly elections. The stakes were very high for the ruling party, which had aggressively campaigned in each of these five states, especially West Bengal. On a normal counting day, the BJP headquarters would be awash with hundreds of journalists, camerapersons, political leaders, party workers and catering staff. But I was astonished to see that the ruling party's national headquarters was completely deserted. There was not a single political leader or party worker there. Not a single newspaper reporter was visible. There were just four television media units stationed outside to do live broadcasts on BJP's prospects as counting progressed. Security guards told us they had strict orders not to allow any individual inside the sprawling multistoried building.

As we patiently waited outside and debated the counting trends, I got a call from my news editor. A children's hospital in south Delhi had just tweeted that it was running out of medical oxygen supply and had stock which would only last a couple of hours. I was told to rush to the Madhukar Rainbow Children's Hospital immediately with my camera unit. This was yet another instance of the oxygen crisis, which was threatening the lives of critical patients on ICU support. By the time I reached the Rainbow hospital, Aam Aadmi Party (AAP) leader Gaurav Chadha had tweeted that he was rushing five oxygen cylinders to meet the emergency needs of critical patients in the children's hospital. After two hours of anxiety, a Delhi Transport Corporation (DTC) bus finally arrived with 10 oxygen cylinders.[39] A few days earlier too, the same hospital had tweeted an SOS for oxygen. It was symptomatic of the oxygen crisis in a large number of hospitals in Delhi-NCR region during the second wave of the COVID-19 pandemic.

The oxygen crisis in many states in April–May 2021 became the defining image of the second wave of COVID-19 pandemic. The unprecedented rise in COVID infection cases in a span of just two to three weeks created an unparalleled humanitarian and health crisis in India. It exposed the fragility of the existing healthcare system in the country. As COVID patients struggled for hospital beds and the scramble for oxygen cylinders intensified, it showed how unprepared India was to fight this pandemic. A large number of patients died because of lack of oxygen. It was one of the worst health crisis in post-independence India.

As the oxygen crisis deepened, the government responded with the largest ever mobilisation of medical oxygen from important industrial centres to augment the growing demand for oxygen from hospitals and COVID care centres. More than 32,000 MT of liquid medical oxygen was transported by 'oxygen express' trains alone by 17 June 2021.[40] Prime Minister Narendra Modi held a series of meetings with chief ministers and district officials to guide them in addressing the oxygen crisis. Under PM-CARES Fund, the Prime Minister's Office sanctioned for the setting up of a total of 1,213 Pressure Swing Adsorption (PSA) oxygen plants to augment oxygen supply in district headquarters and tier-II cities. The prime minister also sanctioned from the PM-CARES Fund the procurement of 1 lakh portable oxygen concentrators.[41]

Desiderata: A New National Law to Fight a Pandemic

India's battle against the COVID-19 pandemic since January 2020 has exposed the fault lines in its governance framework to combat such a public health disaster in future. The COVID-19 pandemic has exposed structural weaknesses in India's emergency governance, public health infrastructure and crisis communication systems. The pandemic has posed complex institutional challenges for every institution/enterprise—both in the government and the private sector. This pandemic occurring once in a century has exposed structural weaknesses in our response mechanism, as every institution has struggled to adapt to the challenges it has posed. The media/social media institutions have a central role to play in setting up an efficacious crisis communication protocol at district, state and national levels.

The media's coverage during the peak of the first coronavirus wave was largely centred on the critical shortage of hospital beds, the debilitating impact of a stringent nationwide lockdown on the economy, especially on the poor and underprivileged people, the reverse migration by more than 11 million migrant workers employed in industrial centres to their home states and an unprecedented rise in unemployment in both urban and rural areas. During the second COVID-19 wave, the critical shortage of ICU beds, essential medicines and medical oxygen in hospitals/COVID care centres, the COVID vaccination-related controversies—both shortage and its slow pace especially from 1 May 2021 onwards when the age restrictions were relaxed and people in the 18–44 years age group were allowed to be vaccinated—dominated the media coverage.

In the wake of the serious governance challenges that India faced, the COVID-19 crisis has highlighted the urgent need for a legislative framework in the form of a new national law to combat the COVID-19-like pandemic in future. The proposed legislation should include a legal framework to set up a national crisis communication protocol and a new framework for health governance. The absence of a viable national crisis communication protocol aggravated the COVID crisis during both the COVID waves. This has necessitated the need to formulate a national crisis communication policy at district, state and national levels to deal with such public health disasters in future. Also, the COVID-19 pandemic has exposed the weaknesses in the existing public health communication systems and highlighted the urgent need to restructure and reform them to meet the challenge posed by such public health disasters in future. Such a policy response would help strengthen the existing public health communication systems.

During a public health disaster, the dissemination of credible information in society is directly proportional to the freedom and the access journalists have to gather news/information and critical data from ground zero. Attempts to 'condition' the newsgathering processes can distort the natural news flow, which is critical in such a crisis situation. As India grapples with one of the biggest public health disasters in its history since the

Spanish flu of 1918–1919, it is also imperative for both the government and the media institutions to strictly implement the goals specified in section 36 (D) of the Sendai Framework for Disaster Risk Reduction 2015–30, which calls for:

> Media to take an active and inclusive role at the local, national, regional and global levels in contributing to the raising of public awareness and understanding and disseminate accurate and non-sensitive disaster risk, hazard and disaster information…in close cooperation with national authorities; adopt specific disaster risk reduction communications policies; support, as appropriate, early warning systems and life-saving protective measures; and stimulate a culture of prevention and strong community involvement in sustained public education campaigns and public consultations at all levels of society, in accordance with national practices.[42]

6

Agriculture in the Time of COVID Pandemic

A Beacon of Hope

HIMANSHU SHEKHAR MISHRA

It was 5 April, the twelfth day after an unprecedented 21-day nationwide lockdown was imposed from the midnight of 24–25 March 2020. India was learning to cope with the worst public health disaster the world had seen since the Spanish influenza pandemic of 1918–1919. With more than a billion people staying indoors, it was perhaps the largest nationwide lockdown in India's post-independence history. Almost all industrial operations, business activities, markets and shopping complexes and air, rail and road transport services had come to a grinding halt. All private and public schools, colleges and government offices, barring those providing important essential services, had been closed down.

As a television news correspondent out in the field to gather and broadcast news on the pandemic, I received a WhatsApp message from Union Agriculture Minister Narendra Singh Tomar's office. The agriculture ministry was closed and most of the senior ministerial office staff was working from home. The WhatsApp message contained a short video statement that the agriculture minister had uploaded on his official Facebook page. It said the central government had sent an advisory to all the state governments to amend the Agriculture Produce Marketing Committee (APMC) Act to facilitate the sale of farmers' agricultural produce right at their doorstep. The objective was to allow buyers/traders to go directly to private godowns of farmers and buy their produce.[1] The advisory was aimed at relaxing the existing mandatory norms for Indian farmers to go to the local grain markets (*anaaj mandis*) to sell their farm produce to licensed or legally authorised buyers.

The union government had taken this major policy decision amid growing fears about the impact of a nationwide lockdown and the pandemic on the agriculture sector. It came at a time when hundreds of millions of farmers were in the process of harvesting their rabi crops and getting ready to transport their produce to the local granary markets for selling them. It was an important decision taken at an exceptionally difficult time to provide relief to millions of farmers. The lockdown had imposed stringent restrictions on transport services, making it exceptionally difficult for farmers to transport their produce to the agriculture trading centres and engage licensed traders and buyers to sell their farm produce.

Also, the exodus of migrant agricultural workers from some of the key farming centres, especially in Punjab and Haryana, following severe restrictions imposed on movement of farm labour during the stringent first phase of the lockdown had led to a labour shortage. It had begun to slow down the rabi harvesting and procurement processes in rural India, thereby affecting the agricultural value chain at several levels. The official intervention by the agriculture ministry was essentially aimed at liberalising the existing legal framework to ease the process of buying and selling of farm produce during the COVID-19 pandemic. It was to mark the beginning of a series of legal interventions by the Government of India (GoI) in the midst of the pandemic to reform the existing decades-old agricultural marketing architecture in the country.

First Exemption to Farm Sector during Lockdown

To facilitate uninterrupted rabi harvesting by hundreds of millions of farmers, the central government gave the first exemption during lockdown to farming and allied activities that were getting affected during the first twenty-one-day lockdown. The home ministry issued orders on 28 March 2020, giving exemptions to the following agriculture and allied sector services and core activities:

1. Agencies engaged in procurement of agriculture products, including minimum support prices (MSP) operations.
2. *Mandis* operated by APMC.
3. Farming operations and farm workers in the field.
4. Fertilizer, pesticide and seed manufacturing and packaging units.

5. Intra- and inter-state movement of harvesting and sowing machines.[2]

Two days later, the government decided to extend the existing 2 per cent interest subvention facility to banks and a 3 per cent timely repayment of incentive benefits to farmers until 31 May 2020, on all crop loans upto ₹3 lakh.[3] As the harvesting activities gradually picked up, the government issued advisories to farmers, urging them to take requisite preventive measures such as maintaining social distancing and personal hygiene, mandatory usage of face masks, cleaning implements and machinery to contain the spread of virus in rural India.[4] To enable seamless harvesting operations across the country, the home ministry on 4 April 2020 decided to allow reopening of shops of agricultural machinery and its spare parts and truck repairs on highways to facilitate unhindered transportation of farm produce.[5]

Rise in Unemployment and 'Reverse' Migration

As the government initiated administrative and legal steps to remove bottlenecks and facilitate agricultural activities across inter-state borders, the lockdown had begun to have a debilitating impact on the micro, small and medium enterprises (MSME) sector. With most of the 6.3 crore MSMEs closed and their supply chain network badly crippled and disrupted, the spectre of hunger and unemployment loomed large on the 11.09 crore workforce employed in this sector.[6]

As India watched with horror, a process of 'reverse' migration soon began from India's leading industrial centres. With millions of factories closed and no means of sustenance available, millions of jobless migrant workers, many with their families, began to march on foot to their home districts situated far away from their workplaces amid growing uncertainty about their future. With public transport services suspended across the country, their tragic and painful migration shocked the world. The plight of unemployed workers migrating to their villages on foot became the image of India's COVID-19 crisis in national and international media during the first phase of the lockdown. India helplessly watched shocking images of an unprecedented humanitarian crisis unfold across several states as millions of migrant workers and their families struggled to walk back home. The humanitarian crisis continued for several weeks as the government was compelled to extend the lockdown restrictions to contain the deadly spread of the virus across the country. The empirical data collected by the Centre for Monitoring Indian Economy (CMIE), a research institution that collects and analyses data on Indian economy, showed the unprecedented employment crisis the lockdown had caused by stalling important economic and industrial activities. In his first analytical report on the impact of lockdown on the employment rate since the imposition of lockdown on 24 March 2020, CMIE Managing Director Mahesh Vyas argued that the unemployment rate had reached an unprecedented level of 23.4 per cent in the country.[7]

Unlocking the Power of Agriculture Sector amid Lockdown

As economic activities remained crippled and unemployment levels continued to rise, Mr Tomar called an important meeting via video conference with all the state agriculture ministers on 9 April 2020. The agenda included the initiation of important legal steps to liberalise the APMC Act at the time of the harvesting season and the effective implementation of exemptions granted by the home ministry to all unhindered agricultural operations across the country. After the meeting, the agriculture ministry released details on the follow-up action being initiated by the respective state governments:

> Advisory (has been) issued to State Governments/ UT on 4th April 2020 to facilitate Direct Marketing, enabling direct purchase from the farmers/FPOs/ Cooperatives etc. by Bulk Buyers/Big Retailers/ Processors by limiting regulation under State APMC Act. Several States like Tamil Nadu, Karnataka and Jharkhand have already initiated action on lines of issued advisory.[8]

As states began to initiate steps to facilitate buying and selling of agricultural produce, I sought an appointment with Mr Tomar to get a first-hand perspective on the central government's big push to reform the agriculture sector. I was one of the first TV news journalists who was granted permission to interview the agriculture minister. A brief conversation with Mr Tomar made it amply clear that the government had decided to push a series of reformist policies and legal measures to strengthen the agriculture sector. In an interview to NDTV, the agriculture minister admitted that the supply of vegetables to the *mandis* had been affected during the lockdown and the farmers were distressed as transporting vegetables to the *mandis* was becoming difficult with transport services largely prohibited and interstate borders being sealed.

He went on to outline steps the central government was planning to take to address such bottlenecks and reform the agriculture sector. Mr Tomar told NDTV:

> During the ongoing COVID-19 crisis, to ensure that farmers earn the right price of every single grain they produce, we have told the state governments to utilise the eNAM (National Agriculture Market) platform for buying and selling farm produce. We have also requested the states to free all farm produce for 3 months from the purview of the Mandi Act. I had an interaction with the state agriculture ministers. 80 per cent of the rabi crops have been harvested as of now and only 20 per cent remains to be harvested... I have advised all the state agriculture ministers to legally allow traders to buy agricultural produce directly from the godowns and warehouses of farmers to overcome the bottlenecks caused by lockdown. I am happy that state agriculture ministers have welcomed our idea. The new system is expected to begin on 15 April 2020. I am confident that states would be successful in buying every single grain farmers will produce within the next 90 days.[9]

On 11 April 2020, Prime Minister Shri Narendra Modi pushed this idea a step further during a virtual interaction with the chief ministers of all states. He urged them to initiate steps to reform the APMC Act and suggested a modification of the APMC law to facilitate unhindered sale of farm produce.[10] As states started to lift lockdown restrictions on agriculture and allied activities, they also began to streamline the harvesting and procurement processes. Soon, the official data from the agriculture sector began to lift the government's morale as relaxations given to agriculture and allied activities during lockdown began to show positive results. An agriculture ministry release said on 10 April 2020 that wheat-producing states had already reported 26–33 per cent harvesting against the total sown area. There was more good news to follow in the next 24 hours. The sowing of summer crops was progressing satisfactorily despite the stringent lockdown. Statistics compiled by the ministry showed that the cultivation of the total area under summer crops (that included rice, pulses, coarse cereals and oilseeds) had increased by 11.64 lakh hectares over 2019.[11]

Soon, the government initiated a new consultation process with exporters of agriculture and allied commodities such as rice, fruits, vegetables, seeds, flowers and agricultural machinery. Some of the key issues discussed in this regard were the shortage of supply of raw materials because of the restrictive functioning of agri-grains markets, the challenges in transporting commodities due to the lockdown, the closure of courier services, phyto-sanitary certifications, the challenges in accessing export/import facilities at the ports/yards, etc. The representatives of the food processing industries demanded an immediate approval to partially restart their business operations.[12] The National Kharif Conference was called two days later to take stock of the preparations for initiating the sowing of kharif crops in the shadow of COVID pandemic during the next cropping season. It was decided to fix the target for food grain production in 2020–2021 at a record 298.3 million tonnes. The government informed the kharif conference that against a food grain production target of 291.10 million tonnes in 2019–2020, a higher production of about 292 million tonnes was anticipated largely because of the enhancement of area coverage and productivity of different crops.[13]

A Grain and a Heap of Hope

The good news from the agriculture sector, coupled with overflowing granaries of the Food Corporation of India (FCI), enabled the government to dole out immediate relief to hundreds of millions of struggling poor and the underprivileged migrant workers and their families who had faced the brunt of the lockdown. The government announced distribution of free foodgrains up to five kilograms (kg) wheat or rice and one kilograms of preferred pulses every month for three months to about 800 million (80 crore) poor and underprivileged people under the Pradhan Mantri Garib Kalyan Ann Yojana (PMGKAY). However, the absence of credible data about migrant workers stranded in different states and the fact that a large number of them had no ration cards made them struggle to access free ration under the PMGKAY.

While shooting a ground report in Faridabad industrial area on the unprecedented job crisis following the lockdown, I met a large number of jobless migrant workers from Bihar and Uttar Pradesh who were stranded with no access to food or job. Many had left their ration cards with their families in their home states. Their inability to access the free foodgrains that the central government was giving had exacerbated the acute financial crisis they were facing.[14]

As the migrant workers crisis unfolded in the national and international media, I sought an appointment with the Union Consumer Affairs, Food and Public Distribution Minister Ram Vilas Paswan. He had just resumed work at his ministerial office in Krishi Bhawan, which was briefly closed after the imposition of lockdown. There were restrictions on movement of office staff inside his office. As I entered his office to request him for an interview, Mr Paswan looked very tense and nervous. He bluntly asked me why I was not carrying a long boom microphone to ensure a six-feet distance during the TV interview. He suggested that reporters should always carry long boom mike to keep themselves safe while reporting on the pandemic. He was worried over news reports that a large number of migrant workers stranded across several states were not able to avail the free foodgrains scheme that the government had launched. Mr Paswan urged all the state governments to utilise the funds allocated under both the National

Disaster Relief Fund (NDRF) and the State Disaster Relief Fund (SDRF) to distribute free foodgrain to migrant workers who had no ration cards.[15] The minister also requested the state governments to buy both wheat and rice at subsidised rates under the Open Market Sale Scheme and distribute food free of cost to the migrant workers. Overflowing granaries had emboldened the government's hand during the pandemic. Mr Paswan argued that the FCI had 300 lakh metric tonne of rice and 235 lakh metric tonne stock of wheat in its godowns, though the country needed just 60 lakh tonnes in a month.

'Slivers of Brightness amidst the Gloom'

As the crisis unfolded, it became clear that agriculture was one of the few slivers of hope for the nation. In an important Monetary Policy Statement on 17 April 2020, the RBI Governor Shaktikanta Das outlined the resilience of agriculture and allied activities:

> ...there are a few slivers of brightness amidst the encircling gloom... By April 10, pre-monsoon Kharif sowing had begun strongly, with acreage of paddy—the principal Kharif crop—up by 37 per cent in comparison with the last season... On April 15, the India Meteorological Department (IMD) forecast a normal south-west monsoon for the 2020 season, with rainfall expected to be 100 per cent of the long period average. These early developments bode well for rural demand ...[16]

As millions of migrant workers reached their homes in the hinterlands, the agriculture sector also became a temporary refuge employer for many of them. The media has documented how a large number of Mumbai's famous *dabbawalas* turned towards agriculture for temporary employment as their business was severely hit during the pandemic.The president of the Dabbawala Association Subhash Talekar told *Hindu BusinessLine*:

> About 95 per cent *dabbawalas* who work in Mumbai are from Pune district and majority of them are back in their villages and have resorted to farming. I am sure that most of them would not return to Mumbai if they earn livelihood in the village. COVID-19 has shattered them from within...Why would people migrate to Mumbai to live in slums if they get work in the village?[17]

The emergence of agriculture as the mainstay of India's ability to withstand the economic crisis during the pandemic made it an important component of Atmanirbhar Bharat—a new governance and developmental initiative for a self-reliant India that emerged during the COVID-19 crisis. In his address to the nation on 12 May 2020, the prime minister outlined its broad objective to make India a global hub of manufacturing and reduce dependence on imports by initiating bold reforms measures to make India more self-reliant. Mr Modi categorically said these reforms included supply chain reforms in the agriculture sector.[18]

Just five days later, on 17 May 2020, Union Finance Minister Nirmala Sitharaman announced a big stimulus package to help alleviate the crisis across different sectors. It included an additional allocation of ₹40,000 crore for the Mahatma Gandhi National Rural Employment Guarantee Scheme (MGNREGS) to create around 300 crore person-days of work in rural India. This was aimed at creating work opportunities for millions of poor and jobless migrants who were forced to return to their home state.

Spanish Flu, Mahatma Gandhi and the Poor Monsoon of 1918

A robust sowing of summer and kharif crops, a good harvest during the rabi season, a record stock of food grains in government's granaries and the expectation of an all-time record food production following an above-average rainfall during the south-west monsoon season in the year 2020 strengthened India's ability to cope with the catastrophic impact of the pandemic. With government granaries having a huge surplus of foodgrain stock, the central government could afford to announce free distribution of five kilograms of wheat or rice to about 800 million (80 crore) poor and underprivileged people till November 2021.

However, the scenario was quite different in 1918–1919, when the Spanish flu pandemic hit the world. With an extremely weak health infrastructure and the absence of basic medical and communication facilities, the Spanish flu had wreaked havoc in India, which was under the British rule at that time. The first case of the Spanish flu was registered on 10 June 1918, a day after the first batch of soldiers returned to the Bombay Port after completing combat duty in the First World War. A group of seven sepoys on duty at the Bombay Port were admitted to hospitals with the flu. Within a few weeks, the pandemic began to spread across India. An estimated 12 million to 13 million Indians are feared to have died from the influenza epidemic during 1918–1919. The Census Report of 1921 states that nearly 8.5 million Indians died in registered areas alone, which accounted for three-fourths of the country's total population at that time.[19] On the basis of the data collected during the Spanish flu pandemic, the Census Report of 1921 said:

> The epidemic was especially virulent in the Rajputana and Central India Agencies and in the States of the Punjab, Central Provinces and Bihar and Orissa, while the attack was severe in Kashmir and Mysore and acute in Hyderabad and parts of Baroda. We have no statistics for these areas, at any rate none that are trustworthy, but a rough estimate would put the direct mortality in them, from the disease in 1918 and 1919, at least in the same proportion as in British territory. We thus arrive at a total mortality of between 12 and 13 million for India.[20]

To make matters worse, the south-west monsoon—the lifeline of Indian agriculture—had remained weak throughout the season in 1918, leading to a below-normal rainfall in the agrarian belt. This was to turn catastrophic for India as it was largely an agrarian economy, and the livelihood of millions of farmers and their families depended solely on the farming sector at that time. The weak monsoon compounded the problem of farmers and agricultural workers, as it meant a significant loss of farm income and depleting food stock at a time when the pandemic was spreading like wildfire across the country.

In his annual report in 1920, the Government of India's sanitary commissioner presented official data on monsoon deficiency. The report said:

> The deficiency in the seasonal rainfall was as much as 81 per cent in Sind, 75 per cent in Rajputana West, 70 per cent in Baluchistan, 63 per cent in Gujarat, and about 50 per cent in the United Provinces West, the Punjab, Rajputana East, Central India East, Berar, the Konkan, the Bombay Deccan, Mysore, and Malabar.[21]

The Census Report of 1921 delineates in detail the agrarian crisis that followed a weak and feeble monsoon. The report states that the monsoon of 1918 was 'exceptionally feeble and gave practically no rain after the beginning of September'. Crop failure was reported from Punjab and many parts of central and western India. This led to the declaration of 'food scarcity' in parts of Punjab, United Provinces, Central Provinces, Bombay, Bihar and Orissa. The scale of human tragedy and the devastating impact of the Spanish flu pandemic on common people in British India was so huge that it wiped off the entire natural increase that could have accrued to the population in the previous seven years.[22] The monsoon remained far below normal until the end of 1920. It created a famine-like situation in many parts of India in 1920, including in one district in Bombay, which was one of the worst-affected province during the Spanish flu period.[23]

This crisis led to a large-scale migration of distressed people from rural India to urban areas in search of work and survival. This aggravated the pandemic situation in the country. This was in stark contrast to the pandemic in 2020, which led to an unprecedented 'reverse' migration by millions of workers from leading industrial centres to their respective home districts in rural and semi-rural areas to survive. The impact of the agrarian crisis on Indian economy was so huge that it took four years for India's per capita GDP to recover after the 1918 pandemic.[24] The 1921 Census Report categorically stated that the Indian population grew by just 1.2 per cent in the previous decade to 318.9 million. The corresponding increase was 7.1 per cent in 1911.[25]

The unprecedented humanitarian crisis unleashed by the influenza epidemic during British India's reign coincided with the rise of Mahatma Gandhi as the leader of India's nascent freedom movement. It is significant to note that Gandhiji himself had contracted the Spanish flu during the second wave of the pandemic while he was living in his Sabarmati Ashram in Ahmedabad. His immediate family suffered badly too as his eldest daughter-in-law and his grandson died of the flu. In fact, the Spanish flu had infected many of Gandhiji's followers in his Sabarmati Ashram. British science journalist Laura Spinney, author of the book *Pale Rider:*

The Spanish Flu of 1918 and How It Changed the World, argues that:

> Medics came to give him the benefit of their advice, but he rejected most of it. Many of them remonstrated with him over his vow not to drink milk—the result of his disgust at the practice of *phooka*, in which air is blown forcefully into a cow's vagina to induce her to lactate.[26]

Gandhiji later relented under pressure from doctors and his wife, Kasturba. He was fortunate to have recovered. Thereafter, he wrote to his eldest son, Hiralal:

> Even after we feel that we have recovered, we must continue to take complete rest in bed and have only easily digestible liquid food. So early as on the third day after the fever has subsided many persons resume their work and their usual diet. The result is a relapse. And quite often a fatal relapse.[27]

Gandhiji and his immediate family suffered from the flu at a time when the British colonial administration had failed to contain the spread of it. The storage of doctors and medical staff had complicated the situation on the ground. The consequent administrative void in the middle of the crisis then led to the emergence of small disparate groups of social and grassroots-level activists who came forward to help the suffering people in different parts of British India. The failure of the British administration in containing the spread of the pandemic fuelled anger against the colonial rule. Ms Spinney has cited historical facts to claim that:

> The people who stepped into that [medical] breach tended to be the militants, the grassroot militant activists for independence who had already worked out how to cross caste barriers and work together for a different goal, i.e. independence. Once the pandemic passed, emotion against the British was even higher than it had been before. Secondly, those people were far more united than they had been. And now they came together behind Gandhi. He found that suddenly, he had the grassroots support that he had been lacking until then.[28]

Though questions have been raised recently as to why the Spanish flu pandemic, which killed an estimated 12 million to 13 million people in India, does not figure prominently in the historical accounts of freedom fighters such as Mahatma Gandhi and Jawaharlal Nehru.[29] Ironically, the larger lessons of the Spanish flu and the requisite policy responses which should have followed were not initiated. In fact, India's inability to learn from the humanitarian crisis perpetrated by the Spanish flu in 1918–1919 has considerably weakened its ability to fight the COVID pandemic in 2020.

Agriculture Absorbed the COVID-19 Shock

While a poor monsoon and the consequent famine in parts of rural India considerably weakened India's ability to withstand the debilitating impact of the Spanish flu in 1918, more than 100 years later, an above-normal south-west monsoon season emerged as a beacon of hope for the Indian agriculture sector during the current pandemic. Amidst the economic ruin across sectors during the lockdown, the agriculture sector stood as firm as the ruling establishment, which immediately initiated institutional steps to further strengthen the sector.

The RBI governor categorically said in his Monetary Policy Statement on 22 May 2020:

> Amidst this encircling gloom, agriculture and allied activities have provided a beacon of hope on the back of an increase of 3.7 per cent in foodgrains production to a new record (as per the third advance estimates of the Ministry of Agriculture released on May 15, 2020... By May 10, 2020 up to which latest information is available, Kharif sowing was higher by 44 per cent over last year's acreage. Rabi procurement is in full flow in respect of oilseeds, pulses and wheat, benefiting from the bumper harvest. These developments will support farm incomes, improve the terms of trade facing the farm sector and strengthen food security for the country.[30]

One Nation, One Agriculture Market

As the economic crisis unfolded and the extent of damage caused by the lockdown became more and more apparent, the government decided to initiate a series of reforms in the agriculture sector. In line with the government's decision, the union cabinet approved three crucial ordinances on 3 June 2020, which were ratified by the President of India on 5 June 2020.

The first ordinance was issued to amend the Essential Commodities Act (ECA) to remove important commodities such as pulses, onions, potatoes, cereals, edible oils and oilseeds from the list of essential commodities. This was aimed at giving the farmers freedom to produce and sell these commodities to attract private sector investments in cold storage, warehouses, food processing and exports sectors.

The second ordinance, titled The Farming Produce Trade and Commerce (Promotion and Facilitation) Ordinance, 2020, was aimed at facilitating a barrier-free interstate and intra-state trade in agriculture produce and building an ecosystem where both farmers and traders could freely sell and purchase their farm produce without paying any cess or levy for the sale. It was designed to pave the way for a 'One India, One Agriculture Market' system. The cabinet also approved the third ordinance, titled The Farmers (Empowerment and Protection) Agreement on Price Assurance and Farm Services Ordinance, 2020. This ordinance was aimed at empowering farmers to engage with processors, aggregators, wholesalers, large retailers and exporters on a level-playing field.

These ordinances outlined a new legal framework to reform the agriculture sector. They were essentially aimed at enhancing private investments in the agriculture and allied sectors, removing institutional bottlenecks to give farmers basic freedom to produce and sell their products, eliminating intermediaries and strengthening the supply chain systems by building new cold chains and warehousing infrastructure and bringing new technology to rural India.

A Press Information Bureau (PIB) release said these agriculture reform measures would help transfer the risk of market unpredictability from farmers to sponsors, enable farmers to access modern technology and help reduce the cost of marketing, thereby improving the income of farmers.[31]

These reform measures brought agriculture to the forefront of the national discourse. While addressing the Confederation of Indian Industry's (CII) National Council on 27 July 2020, the RBI governor listed the growing transformation in Indian agriculture as the first of the five dynamic shifts that could shape the future of the Indian economy.[32] The decision to implement the three ordinances was followed by a series of policy measures to increase new investments in agriculture. The prime minister launched a ₹1 lakh crore Agriculture Infrastructure Fund on 9 August 2020, a medium- and long-term debt financing facility for investment in viable projects for post-harvest management infrastructure and community farming assets through an interest subvention and credit guarantee.[33]

Second Corona Wave Hits Rural India

While the agriculture sector emerged as a beacon of hope during the first COVID wave in 2020, the spread of cases in villages and small rural towns during the second corona virus wave became a subject of national concern in April–May 2021. It was shocking when media agencies began to report that unidentified dead bodies had begun to wash up along the banks of the holy river Ganges in Bihar and Uttar Pradesh, India's two most populous states, in the second week of May 2021. There was widespread fear among locals that these dead bodies had been immersed in rivers after families ran out of wood for their cremation.[34] As district administrations began to investigate the case, social media platforms were soon awash with videos and images of dead bodies flowing in rivers, especially in Bihar, UP and Madhya Pradesh. This was followed by widespread fear about the rising COVID cases in villages and rural towns and growing discrepancy between official COVID-19 deaths and actual numbers on the ground. NDTV reported from the Bamhaur Khas village in the Kaimur district situated along the Bihar–UP border on 13 May 2021 that 34 people had lost their lives from COVID-like symptoms in just 25 days and 70 per cent of the residents in this village had fallen ill.[35]

It revived eerie memories of the 1918 Spanish flu when dead bodies in large numbers were dumped in the river Ganges. The leading Hindi poet and writer Shri Suryakant Tripathi 'Nirala' has recorded the incident in his widely read biography *Kulli Bhat* (1938). Niralaji has given a graphic description of the humanitarian tragedy that befell his family and the devastation perpetrated by the Influenza flu in Indian villages. Niralaji wrote,

> There was a violent outbreak of influenza about this time... I received a telegram: "Your wife is gravely ill. Come immediately." I was twenty-two... The newspapers had informed us about the ravages of the epidemic. I travelled to the riverbank in Dalmau and waited. The Ganga was swollen with dead bodies.

> At my in-law's house, I learned that my wife had passed away.[36] (*A Life Misspent*, 2016).

More than a hundred years later, history seemed to be repeating itself. As concern rose over lack of COVID-testing facilities in villages and rural towns and COVID-19 cases continued to rise alarmingly, in a direct online interaction with farmers of several states on 14 May 2021, the prime minister warned them over the threat posed by the rise in COVID infection cases in villages:

> I want all the farmers and brothers and sisters living in villages to remain alert against Corona. This pandemic is spreading fast in rural villages. Every government is taking efforts to meet with this challenge. Awareness about this among rural people and cooperation of the panchayat institutions are equally important... Free vaccination is going on in government hospitals across the country. Therefore, get yourself vaccinated when your turn comes. This will give you protection and reduce the risk of serious illnesses.[37]

The prime minister's warning followed worrying news reports about the disturbing rise in COVID-related deaths in villages of Uttar Pradesh. He followed this up with a series of directives to officials in a COVID review meeting on 15 May 2021 to conduct door-to-door testing in rural areas. A Prime Minister's Office release said:

> PM asked for augmentation of healthcare resources in rural areas to focus on door to door testing &

> surveillance. He also spoke about empowering ASHA & Anganwadi workers with all necessary tools. PM asked for guidelines to be made available in an easy language along with illustrations for home isolation and treatment in rural areas. The prime minister directed that a distribution plan for ensuring oxygen supply in rural areas should be worked out, including through provision of Oxygen Concentrators.[38]

Within 20 hours of the prime minister's directive, the union health ministry issued a standard operating procedure on containment and management of COVID in peri-urban, rural and tribal areas on 16 May 2021. It specifically warned: "A gradual ingress is now being seen in peri-urban, rural and tribal areas as well. In view of this, there is a need to enable communities, strengthen primary level healthcare infrastructure at all levels to intensify COVID-19 response in peri-urban, rural and tribal areas, while continuing to provide other essential health services.'[39] The health ministry's advisory to states was to set up 30-bed COVID Care Centres in peri-urban and rural areas and devise strategies for achieving high coverage with COVID vaccinations in rural areas.

As national concern grew over an alarming increase in COVID cases in rural India, the prime minister choked up during an online interaction with doctors and healthcare workers of Varanasi as he emotionally paid tribute to those who had died. The prime minister said, 'This virus has snatched many of our loved ones from us. I pay my humble tribute to them and I express my condolences to the families who lost people'.[40] He directed that the district administration must give greater attention to rural areas in Varanasi and the Poorvanchal region.

Unemployment Crisis and Rural Poverty

While India struggled to cope with the spread of COVID infections in rural areas, the decision to impose state-wise lockdowns to contain the second wave of COVID-19 pandemic began to cast its dark shadow on the future of economically poor and underprivileged workers and their families. With several state governments forced to impose lockdown and night curfew starting April 2021, it had a debilitating impact on the weakest section of the migrant and unorganised sector workers, who had already suffered a severe loss of income during the stringent nationwide lockdown during the first coronavirus wave in 2020.

Azim Premji University researchers argued in their 'State of Working India 2021' report that the income of around 230 million poor Indian workers fell below the national minimum wage threshold (₹375 per day as recommended by the Anoop Satpathy committee) between March and October 2021. The researchers have argued:

> This amounts to an increase in the poverty rate by 15 percentage points in rural and nearly 20 percentage points in urban areas. Had the pandemic not occurred, poverty would have declined by 5 percentage points in rural areas and

> 1.5 percentage points in urban areas between 2019 and 2020, and 50 million would have been lifted above this line.'[41]

In fact, the impact of the second coronavirus wave on employment was devastating in April 2021. The Centre for Monitoring Indian Economy's Managing Director Mahesh Vyas told me in an interview that an estimated 70 lakh Indian workers had lost their jobs in April 2021 alone. This included around 28 lakh salaried workers and 6 lakh daily wage labourers.[42] The MSME sector was one of the worst affected. The national president of Clothing Manufacturers Association of India, Rajesh Masand, told me in an interview that 77 per cent MSMEs engaged in the garment manufacturing sector were planning to cut staff strength by more than 25 per cent if the uncertainty lengthens.[43]

As the period of lockdown lengthened, the unemployment crisis began to deepen. The Centre for Monitoring Indian Economy's (CMIE) data on unemployment rate in the week ending 16 May 2021 showed that unemployment at the all-India level had risen to 14.45 per cent, with urban unemployment rate reaching 14.71 per cent and rural unemployment levels reaching 14.34 per cent. In the previous week ending 9 May 2021, the unemployment rate in the country was 8.67 per cent with urban unemployment rate at 11.72 per cent and rural unemployment at just 7.29 per cent.[44] The data showed that the state-wise partial and full lockdown imposed had aggravated the unemployment crisis in the country, in both urban and rural India.

As economic activities got hindered, it was the poor and migrant workers who had to face the brunt of lockdown like the first COVID-19 wave which had witnessed large-scale 'reverse' migration in 2020. Significantly, the suspension of work under India's largest employment generation scheme—Mahatma Gandhi Rural Employment Guarantee Scheme (MGNREGS)—during the lockdown aggravated the situation on the ground. We shot a ground report in Sonbhadra District of Uttar Pradesh which showed how the local administration had stopped all work under Mahatma Gandhi National Rural Employment Guarantee Act (MGNREGA) thereby aggravating the misery of poor villagers and migrant workers. A 42-year-old migrant worker Indradev Prasad told us he worked in a private company in Gorakhpur. After losing his job last year during the first wave of the pandemic during the nationwide lockdown, he had returned to his village. Initially, he managed to get work for 50 days under MGNREGA. But the imposition of lockdown had led to the stoppage of all work under MGNREGA in May 2021, leading to acute financial distress for his family.

The Kewal village Gram Sewak Ramchandra told NDTV, 'Before 28 April 2021, 120 to 130 villagers used to get work under MGNREGA, which has stopped now. We have no alternative means of social security. There is no work available for us now.'[45] The problem for resident villagers has become complicated because of the delay in the release of payment for the work done before the lockdown. Kewal village resident 30-year-old Urmila Devi got work for 40 days with her husband in the construction of a *baoli* (stepwell) in the village under MGNREGA. But Urmila told NDTV that the payment has not yet been released. She said, 'We worked under MGNREGA. The *munshi* told us to check our bank account. But the money has not reached my bank account.' Gram Pradhan Dinesh Yadav said many migrant workers have returned to the village after losing jobs. They are facing financial duress.

As the employment crisis rose in villages, the union rural development ministry issued data which said that despite the COVID crisis, 1.85 crore people were offered work in May 2021 under MGNREGA. The work offered was 52 per cent higher than that offered during the same period in May 2019, where 1.22 crore people were paid under the scheme per day. This increase was recorded despite casualties either through death or infection among the operating staff at all levels, including those on the front line. The significant rise in the work demanded under MGNREGA reflected the growing demand and search for work among the poor and migrant workers.

7

Migration and Food Security during the Pandemic

An Acid Test for Government Policies

RABINDRANATH BHATTACHARYYA

When this chapter was initiated, migrant labourers across the country were walking back in droves to their villages from cities thousands of kilometres away due to the pandemic-induced lockdown. The situation was completely out of control. There was no SOP that could be followed to mitigate the hunger of a grossly estimated (no one knows the exact number even today) eight crore migrant population whose livelihoods had been suddenly snatched away. The government response was debatable and the media questioned it relentlessly. After the first wave of the pandemic, the home ministry apprised the Parliamentary Standing Committee on Home Affairs (Report No. 229 on 'Management of COVID-19 Pandemic and Related Issues', presented to the chairman, Rajya Sabha, on 21 December 2020) that 'India adopted a proactive, pre-emptive and graded response to deal with the unprecedented global crisis declared as a "pandemic" by the World Health Organization'. But the second wave that started in India in mid-February 2021 washed away all these 'pro-active, pre-emptive and graded responses.' Since the end of the first week of May 2021, the second wave is declining, although the scary Delta+ variant and Omicron variant of the virus are looming large and black fungus or Mucormycosis has already been declared as an epidemic in Tamil Nadu, Odisha, Gujarat and UT of Chandigarh under the Epidemic Diseases Act, 1897.[1] Despite the lessons learnt, the experiences acquired in this period regarding migration have shaken the written memory of an epidemic in India.

Jyoti Kumari, a 15-year-old daughter of a migrant worker from the Sirhulli village in Bihar's Darbhanga district, hit the headlines for the way she helped her father during the lockdown. Her father, a migrant e-rickshaw puller, broke a leg due to an accident in Gurugram, Haryana. Jyoti travelled from the village to look after her father and be with him in January 2020. After the extended lockdown was declared to contain the spread of the coronavirus, Jyoti and her father lost their source of income. After being told by their landlord to vacate their rented room, Jyoti cycled more than 1,200 kilometres in seven days to take her injured father back to their village in Bihar. (Unfortunately, he passed away after a cardiac arrest on 31 May 2021.) Watching the news on television, the then US President Donald Trump's daughter Ivanka Trump, who was also his senior advisor, tweeted encouraging words about Jyoti's 'beautiful feat of endurance and love'. Jyoti's is just one of the many stories of the suffering of millions of migrant labourers, who were almost invisible to the *bhadraloks* of India before the lockdown was declared throughout India at just four hours' notice.

From 26 March 2020, various journals, blogs on human rights, websites and news media channels began to publish reports of the plight of the stranded and out-of-work interstate migrant labourers, many of whom died due to train or road accidents or simply out of hunger on their long journey back home. In some cases, they travelled a distance of 1,500 kilometres.[2]

A pregnant migrant labourer was walking back from Nashik, Maharashtra, to her village in Satna, Madhya Pradesh, 1,100 kilometres away. On the way back, she gave birth, rested for just two hours and then resumed the walk for another 150 kilometres to reach Satna. It was only after reaching there that she was taken to a hospital by the local authorities.[3]

On 21 May 2020, journalist Shagun Kapil reported in *Down to Earth*, an online news journal, that a land and forest rights organisation Ekta Parishad had interviewed 31,423 migrants (till 20 May 2020) to know whether they wanted to return home or stay back at their places of work. They found that 95 per cent of migrant workers preferred to return home despite the threat of financial insecurity and unemployment thereafter.

The narrative had many different versions. Some states made arrangements for those who were coming back home. Quarantine centres would provide meals and essential items, such as mosquito nets and/or sanitisers, but in most parts of the country, migrant labourers were seen as carriers of COVID and were not even allowed to enter their villages. On 29 May 2020, *Hindustan Times* reported the story of an agricultural worker who rode almost 900 kilometres in a motorcycle from Delhi to his home, only to be denied entry into his village.[4]

In another such story, seven migrant labourers from the Bhangidih village of Purulia in West Bengal were left with no choice but to stay for a week on trees to protect themselves from the attack of wild elephants. The labourers had returned from Chennai, but there were no quarantine centres for them in the village and their families lived in a single-room *kuccha* hut in the village. So they couldn't stay in isolation at home either.[5]

Then, from the first week of June 2020 as the unlocking began, some migrants began another journey to return to their workplaces. This time, too, there were no train services available, as the railway ministry had decided to keep services suspended.

Moved by all the suffering that India's poorest were going through, lyricist Gulzar penned an emotional poem in Hindi that reflected the ultimate wishes of the migrant labourers. It said: 'If I have to die, I will die going there, where there is life.'

Between 24 June 2020 and 8 July 2020, a survey was conducted by the Aga Khan Rural Support Programme (India) in association with some other non-government organisations, titled 'How is the Hinterland Unlocking?' The survey covered 4,835 households in 48 districts of 11 states. It was found that almost one-third of the migrants who had walked home to their villages were now back in the cities. Half of them who were still in villages wanted to return.[6]

Then the second wave started in mid-February 2021. On 4 April 2021, the number of COVID infections surpassed the previous peak. On 14 April 2021, it rose above 2 lakh.[7] That day, Maharashtra declared a lockdown once again, but not as stringent as the national lockdown of 2020. Delhi, too, declared lockdown on 19 April. Gradually other states also followed suit. The situation for the migrant workers went back to what it was in 2020. On 13 May 2021, the Supreme Court of India made a query to the central government as well as the Delhi, Uttar Pradesh and Haryana governments regarding their plans on delivering relief to the migrant workers who remained stranded in those states due to the lockdown.[8] The Supreme Court directed the authorities to deliver ration to migrants on self-declaration and not insist on an identity card. However, this did not help the migrants much since they still had no jobs and their savings had already been exhausted.[9]

This begs the question: Why did the migrants then bear such hardship to return to their villages in the first place? Why did they endure the chaos and the gross violation of human rights? Then why did they come back to their places of work again? Should society and the people, who are reaping benefits of migrant labour, allocate a permanent place for them to dwell in the cities? Finally, why should people have to migrate at all?

India's Migrant Workers

Interstate migration and quarantine are on Item 81 of the Seventh Schedule (Union List) of the Indian constitution. The International Organization for

Migration (IOM) defines a migrant as 'a person who moves away from his or her place of usual residence, whether within a country or across an international border, temporarily or permanently, and for a variety of reasons'.[10] To ensure food security through employment is one of the main reasons why people migrate from one part to another within the country or outside. In all developing countries, people migrate from one district to another or from one state to another or even outside the country in search of economic opportunities and jobs so that poverty and hunger can be avoided.

In January 2017, the Ministry of Housing and Urban Poverty Alleviation prepared a report of the working group on migration. It was observed that: 'Data from the National Sample Survey (NSS) in 2007–2008 (the limited available data from Census 2011 does not include workers) reveals that about 28.3% of the workforce in India are migrants.'[11] The report, however, does not mention the actual number of internal migrant labourers in India.

According to a report of the World Bank Group KNOMAD, 'The number of internal migrants is about two-and-a-half times that of international migrants. China and India each have over 100 million internal migrants.'[12] According to the KNOMAD report, the lockdown, travel ban and social distancing led to an agonising process of reverse migration in India and in many Latin American countries.[13]

The situation in India becomes complex because of the invisibility of the interstate migrant workers. In volume I of the *Economic Survey 2018–19* (two volumes) released on 4 July 2019, it was noted: 'Therefore, with

93 percent workers in the informal economy, a well-designed minimum wage system can reduce inequalities in incomes, bridge gender gaps in wages and alleviate poverty.'[14] The actual number of workers remaining in the informal economy has not been mentioned. Migrant workers mostly work on the basis of an informal nature of contract, 'providing transitional form of living and livelihood for them'.[15] So the government does not have an idea of the exact number of migrants in each state and their identification status, which is the real problem for delivering social security. Also, well-governed migratory processes lead to far more target-oriented substantial contributions to the economic and social development of a country. However, India doesn't have a national register for migrant labourers, whether internal or international. As a result, there is no labour code on occupational safety and health and working condition of the migrant workers. Instead, there is a large unorganised sector of contractors (*thekedars*) who mobilise the labourers for work. In the process, both the *thekedars* and the project developers reap profits.

It is true that the new millennium has been marked by increasing informalisation of markets due to a lack of adequate job opportunities. However, that should be supplemented by rights-based distributive policies from the government so that workers in the unorganised sector are not exploited by the employers.

Besides, the unorganised sector in India is divided and sub-divided into many types of regular and casual contracts by divergent labour processes, such as contracting out and home-working, and by social stratification and inequity in accordance with various categories of identity. The categories are native place, caste, ethnic origin, religion, gender, seniority status and state of health. This makes it very hard to organise the migrant workers.[16] These kind of complex discriminations in contractual obligations cutting across native place, caste, ethnic origin, religion and gender cannot be resolved by any policy measures unless there are some non-policy remedies such as bringing organisations or individuals together with the help of some voluntary organisations to work on the issue.

'Without Any Cash or Work, How Will I Survive?'

That was the first question that came to Ram Kewat's mind after he walked 450 kilometres from Delhi to his home on the outskirts of Jhansi. Kewat is a 60-year-old daily wage labourer from Delhi.[17] He was just one of the millions of labourers.

In Uttarakhand alone, at least 550 villages had lost half of their population to migration, so much so that they began to be referred as *bhootiya gaon* or ghost villages.[18] With reverse migration during the first wave of the pandemic, these villages came back to life.

The data provided by the Centre for Monitoring Indian Economy (CMIE) revealed that the rate of workforce that remained unemployed in India in March 2020 was 8.8 per cent. The same rate in April 2020 rose to 23.52 per cent.[19]

Migrant workers in India faced certain loss of entitlement to resources during the pandemic that could enable them to have a secure life. The media narratives on the migrant workers focused on the single point that the imposition of the sudden lockdown had made them jobless, cashless, homeless and foodless. To seek refuge from this unprecedented uncertainty, they all chose to walk thousands of kilometres.

On 28 May 2020, the Solicitor General of India, on behalf of the union government, intimated the Supreme Court that from 1 May 2020 onwards, 97 lakh migrant workers went back to their native places. Of which, 5 million migrants had returned home by train and 4.1 million by road. In a written response to a question posed by the opposition in the Lok Sabha on 14 September 2020, the labour ministry intimated that it did not have any data on migrants' death and hence the 'question does not arise' for any compensation.[20] However, *Hindustan Times* reported on 2 June 2020 that until then 198 migrant workers had lost their lives on their way back home due to accidents or other reasons.[21]

On 9 June 2020, the Supreme Court issued three very important directives. It said:

1. All States and UTs would mandatorily identify stranded migrants and transport them back to their hometowns within 15 days.
2. States must consider withdrawal of all lockdown violations-related cases against migrants under Disaster Management Act.
3. The railways should provide *shramik* trains within 24 hours, if there was a demand.

One Nation, One Ration Card

From this, it is understood that the migrant workers required food security and cash for paying house rent and other fixed establishment expenses. For ensuring a flexible food supply chain and a seamless public distribution system (PDS), on 14 May 2020, the finance minister declared the launch of a One Nation One Ration Card (ONORC) system for ration card holders across the country. The concept of ONORC has changed the concept of food security in the country. ONORC maintains that a person is entitled to draw his/her ration from anywhere in India. Such a system needs digitisation of ration cards, which is difficult to be implemented in a country like ours. As per the announcement of the Ministry of Finance on 11 March 2021, 17 states have successfully implemented ONORC.[22] Also, on 11 June 2021, the Supreme Court observed that states and union territories must implement ONORC, so that the migrant workers may get their rations in states where they are not registered.[23]

The second policy that was launched by the prime minister on 30 June 2020 was the Feed India Mission. Under this, it was decided that all marginal sections of the population would be given free food for six months until 30 November 2020. This included the liberally estimated 8 crore migrant workers under the Atmanirbhar Bharat scheme. On 7 June 2021, the prime minister, in his televised speech to the nation, again promised a fixed quantity of free foodgrains to be made available to 800 million citizens till Diwali, that is, 4 November 2021. Together, these two policies of the central government were supposed to ensure zero hunger in a sustainable manner in the aftermath of the lockdown.

On 2 July 2020, the Ministry of Consumer Affairs, Food and Public Distribution posted a statement on the PIB website that said that under the Atmanirbhar Bharat scheme, the government wanted to target about 8 crore migrant persons (10 per cent of total 80 crore National Food Security Act beneficiaries) for the allocation of 4 lakh metric tonnes of foodgrains per month for a period of two months, that is, in May and June 2020. On 30 June 2020, this period was extended to six months under the Prime Minister's Feed India Mission. Despite these policies, the situation was not as promising as expected in the post-pandemic era and food security could not be ensured for the marginalised. On 21 May 2021, as reported in *The News Minute*, the Karnataka High Court, based on the application of the People's Union for Civil Liberties (PUCL), wanted the state government to ensure food security through universal allocation of foodgrains and health packets to be delivered at doorsteps without insisting on ration cards.[24]

Food for Thought

Food security thrives on three pillars in any country: availability, affordability and accessibility of foodgrains. The availability of foodgrains depends on their production and creating and maintaining a buffer stock. The affordability and accessibility, on the other hand, depend on the distribution system of a country.

In the report on 'The State of Food Security and the Nutrition of the World 2020', the UN Food and Agricultural Organization (FAO) noted that the sustainable goal of zero hunger had taken a hit after the pandemic, with a substantial increase in the number of undernourished people throughout the world. According to the report, 'In 2019, close to 750 million—or nearly one in ten people in the world—were exposed to severe levels of food insecurity.'[25] The situation is so dire now that there will be an increase of 10 million hungry people in the ensuing year and 60 million people in five years. This severe food insecurity will lead to a decline in the quality and quantity of food that marginalised people consume.[26]

A substantial number of those hungry people will be from India. Although India has a large amount of available food stock, it remains a very poor performer, as indicated in the Global Hunger Index (GHI). According to the GHI Report 2021, India ranks 101 among 116 countries with a score of 27.5. In 2020, India scored 27.2 and ranked 94 among 107 countries, while in 2019 India scored 30.3 and ranked 102 among 117 countries. According to the GHI Severity Scale, a score of 20–34.9 indicated a serious situation. This shows that even before the pandemic hit, the hunger situation in India was quite grim.

Unlike developed countries, food security in India is counted in terms of availability of cereals such as rice, wheat and pulses. It does not include meat, milk, fruit or other luxury items. Data provided by the Directorate of Economics and Statistics, Ministry of Agriculture and Farmers Welfare, Government of India (2017), shows that the total foodgrain production in India has consistently increased (except for the years 2014–2015 and 2015–2016) from 50.8 million tonnes in 1950–1951 to 275.1 million tonnes in 2016–2017[27] although the percentage distribution of gross cropped area for total foodgrains has consistently decreased from 76.7 in 1950–1951 to 62.3 in 2014–2015.[28] It has been widely reported in the news media[29] that India was estimated to touch an all-time high foodgrain production of 295.67 million tonnes in the 2019–2020 crop year.

On the other hand, as per the foodgrain stock in the central pool for the year 2020 (as seen on the Food Corporation of India website), total available stock of rice was 322.39, 285.03 and 274.44 lakh metric tonnes in the months of April, May and June 2020, respectively. Moreover, for wheat it was 247.00, 357.70 and 558.25 lakh metric tonnes, respectively. This is a huge stock, which, if properly distributed, could really help achieve zero hunger.

Inefficient Public Delivery System

On 8 July 2020, *India Today* reported the horror story of sexual torture of tribal minor girls by contractors and middlemen of illegal mines 'in exchange for a few morsels of food and some money' at Chitrakoot in the Bundelkhand region of Uttar Pradesh. As narrated by those girls, 'The double whammy of poverty and the months-long lockdown has hit them hard and made them far more vulnerable to exploitation.'[30] One of the girls' mother said they did not have work for three months and consequently they were running from pillar to post to get a square meal a day for the family.[31] This is significant since it reveals that those tribal families of Chitrakoot neither got the benefits under the Pradhan Mantri Garib Kalyan Yojana or of the Direct Benefit Transfer in their Jan-Dhan accounts.

In view of the unavailability of data on migrants and the absence of digitised ration cards during the first wave of the pandemic (essential in the integrated management of PDS), the distribution of foodgrains became a huge problem. Thus, it was found that although 6.39 lakh metric tonnes of foodgrains were procured by the states and the UTs for the months of May and June 2020, they distributed only 99,207 metric tonnes among 209.96 lakh beneficiaries (120.08 lakh in May and 89.88 lakh in June).[32] So, among the government-estimated 8 crore beneficiaries, only 2.996 crore could receive the foodgrains. Thus, although the foodgrain was available and the government had intended to distribute it among marginalised people for free, that did not happen.

An efficient PDS ensures that the targeted distribution of foodgrains fulfils its objective and nobody is excluded from food support. If migrant labourers do not have ration cards, it will not be possible for any government official to distribute food to them until there is a court order because in the future they will be liable to a government audit. So, ration cards are a must for providing food security by a government network. Accessibility of entitlement through ONORC may again be a problem, as it has been conceived on the biometric system of Aadhaar cards and the networks still remain very weak in remote areas of India. This may lead to exclusion of some of the most vulnerable sections from getting social security entitlement. Thus, authentication of need on the basis of identity remains a major bottleneck for the procedural accountability of the institutions of PDS.

In December 2016, NITI Aayog, a public policy think tank of GoI, published a report[33] on the Evaluation Study on Role of Public Distribution System in Shaping Household and Nutritional Security in India. Some of the basic points for the inefficiency of PDS noted in the key findings there were:

1. Bureaucratic difficulties, which was viewed as being 'the single most important reason for households not having a card'.
2. High inclusion and exclusion errors.
3. Highest exclusion errors among marginalised groups.

One of the major reasons of the error of exclusion from the list of beneficiaries of the National Food Security Act (NFSA) 2013 was that the beneficiaries were identified on the basis of the decade-old census of 2011.

In 2018, Rupayaan, an NGO in Odisha that was working on food and nutrition issues, noted that the simple rule of aggregating ST and SC population data in the state by ignoring multiple deprivation factors such as migration at the district level had been another major reason for the exclusion of the beneficiaries from NFSA.[34] They also suggested that the practice of positive discrimination of giving priority in allotment of food to underdeveloped areas at the state, district and sub-district levels may be important for suitable inclusion of the beneficiaries in the state.[35] These recommendations can be imbibed by other states as well.

Populism Versus Welfare-Consequentialism

It is often said that public policy in developing countries like India, unlike the developed ones, are mainly guided by populism that arises from typically not-so-well-educated people.

Populism as a social and political phenomenon contains four key ideas:

1. Presence of two distinct groups: the people and the established elite.
2. Between whom a contradictory relationship exists.
3. In this relationship, the people are considered as righteous and the elite are besmirched.
4. The popular will remains the root of legitimacy.[36]

Populism claims that public policy will be the articulation of *volonte generale* (general will) of the people.[37]

On the other hand, consequentialism identifies the goodness of any act as the goodness of the expected outcomes.[38] Welfare can be measured objectively such as by an increase in health, education or income indicators or subjectively by the perception of people regarding government activities. The analysis of the migrant mayhem and food security in India during the pandemic brought us to a situation where policy formulation reflected populism. However, welfare consequentialism fails in the targeted delivery of services of PDS or delivering social justice to the internal migrants from the perspective of expected outcomes. Let us examine why it is so.

In India, populism in public policy per se is reflected through the responsive policy formulation rather than a proactive one. India possesses a multicultural society containing diverse ethnic groups, linguistic communities, religious identities and caste groups. In such a society, the central government, even with a strong majority, is cautious about being proactive in formulating a policy until it is strongly bonded to the ideology of the ruling party, so that the formulated policy does not become a political issue for the opposition parties.

In case of the migrant workers, the situation remains more complex, as it is well known that they provide development to the host region but send their remittances to their native places. This leads to pressure groups in the host region demanding restrictive policies regarding migrant workers. So, the host states ignore central labour legislations on informal workers. On the other hand, the state authorities of the native places often ignore the social security rights of the migrant workers as they do not contribute to development there. Thus, migrant workers remain 'job thieves' to the local people of the host state and 'disloyal' to the native state. Hence, responsive policy formulation towards migrants shows a lack of a rational choice in identifying the problem as well as defining and ranking goals, considered to be the first two stages in the traditional top-down policy formulation process.[39]

One basic reason of this short-sightedness in the policy formulation process is the lack of decentralised feedback in policy formulation. It is well known that the Prime Minister's Office (PMO) has become more centralised, specifically since the second term of Prime Minister Narendra Modi. Former Union Home Secretary G.K. Pillai was reported[40] to have described the PMO, during Modi's second term, as even more powerful compared to the first term with centralised power and viewed that it would continue to be so. Identifying all policy alternatives and choosing the best among them for policy formulation ultimately rests with the PMO, and if they miss the right information, it would be disastrous.

Public Morality—Need of the Hour

The problems migrants face are largely due to the presence of an unorganised and informal sector in the country. Identification of the migrant workforce on the basis of biometric authentication will have a direct impact on food security as well as on targeted PDS.

Theodore Lowi identified the making of policy as 'an act of setting a public morality upon some action or status hitherto considered private'.[41] Lowi also classified redistributive public policy as one of the four types of public policy, which ensures social security. Of course, that is done by redistributing resources from one group to another.

The entire analysis of this chapter shows that the formulation of redistributive policy on the basis of a 'public morality' in India is determined by populist politics, whereas the benefits of those policies are limited by institutional complexities. The aim is to locate the policy conditions empirically rooted in political patterns. If we do that, we are bound to get better implementation of policies as well as improved delivery of services, be it for securing social justice for migrant workers or for ensuring food security for all vulnerable and marginalised sections of society.

References

Dutta, Anisha. 2020. '198 Migrant Workers Killed in Road Accidents during Lockdown: Report', *Hindustan Times*, 2 June, https://www.hindustantimes.com/india-news/198-migrant-workers-killed-in-road-accidents-during-lockdown-report/story-hTWzAWMYnokyycKw1dyKqL.html, accessed 17 October 2020.

Economic Survey 2018–19, Ministry of Finance, Department of Economic Affairs, Economic Division, Government of India, July 2019, Vol. 1, https://www.indiabudget.gov.in/budget2019-20/economicsurvey/index.php.

'Exploring Cash Transfer to Jan Dhan Accounts as COVID-19 Response: Findings from A Rapid Survey (28 April to 12 May 2020) for Assessing the Ground Reality', National Coalition of Civil Society Organization, May 2020, https://www.oxfamindia.org/sites/default/files/2020-06/Rapid%20Survey-Cash%20Transfer%20to%20Jan%20Dhan%20Account%20Holders-Report-26%20May%20202....pdf.

'Food grains Stock in Central Pool for the years 2016-2020', Food Corporation of India, http://fci.gov.in/stocks.php?view=46,accessed 21 July 2020.

Harriss-White, Barbara, and ValentinaProsperi. 2014. 'The Micro Political Economy of Gains by Unorganised Workers in India', *Economic and Political Weekly*, 1 March.

International Migration Law-Glossary on Migration, International Organization for Migration, UN, Geneva, 2019.

Jha, Prashant and Ishita Mishra. 2020. 'Uttarakhand's "Ghost Villages" Spring Back to Life', *Times of India*, 17 June, http://timesofindia.indiatimes.com/articleshow/76412902.cms?utm_source=contentofinterest&utm_medium=text&utm_campaign=cppst, accessed 21 July 2020.

Lowi, Theodore, J. 1972. 'Four Systems of Policy, Politics and Choice', *Public Administration Review*, Vol. 32, No. 4 (Jul. - Aug.), 298–310.

Mathur, Kuldeep. 2013. *Public Policy and Politics in India - How Institutions Matter*. New Delhi, Oxford University Press.

Migration and Development Brief 32, KNOMAD, World Bank Group, April 2020, https://www.knomad.org/sites/default/

files/2020-06/R8_Migration%26Remittances_brief32.pdf, accessed10 June 2020.

Ministry of Consumer Affairs, Food & Public Distribution. 2020. 'Under AtmaNirbhar Bharat Scheme, Intended Target of 8 Crore Migrant Persons (10% of Total 80 crore NFSA Beneficiaries) was Estimated; Allocation of 4 LMT Foodgrains Per Month was Made@10% of Monthly Allotment under NFSA for Free Distribution', PIB, 2 July, https://pib.gov.in/PressReleasePage.aspx?PRID=1635952.

Mondal, P. 2020. 'Walked from Chennai to West Bengal, Seven Migrants Self-Isolate on Trees to Protect Family from COVID-19', *New Indian Express*, 29 March, https://www.newindianexpress.com/thesundaystandard/2020/mar/29/walked-from-chennai-to-west-bengal-seven-migrants-self-isolate-on-trees-to-protect-family-from-covid-19-2122800.html.

Pocket Book of Agricultural Statistics, Directorate of Economics & Statistics, Ministry of Agriculture & Farmers Welfare, Government of India, 2017, New Delhi, http//:agricoop.nic.in/sites/default/files/pocketbook 0.pdf, as accessed on 21 July2020

PTI. 2020. 'India's Foodgrains Production to Touch Record 295.67 MT in 2019–20 Crop Year', *Financial Express*, 15 May 2020, https://www.financialexpress.com/economy/indias-foodgrains-production-to-touch-record-295-67-mt-in-2019-20-crop-year/1960151/, accessed 21 July 2020.

PTI. 2020. 'Govt Projects 4th Consecutive Year of Record Foodgrain Output at 295.67 Million Tonnes for 2019-20', *Firstpost*, 15 May 2020, https://www.firstpost.com/business/govt-projects-4th-consecutive-year-of-record-foodgrain-output-at-295-67-million-tonnes-for-2019-20-8371631.html, accessed 21 July 2020.

'Report of the Working Group On Migration', Ministry of Housing and Urban Poverty Alleviation, Government of India 2017.

Semple, Noel. 2020. 'Welfare-Consequentialism: A Vaccine for Populism?' *The Political Quarterly*, Wiley Online Library, 1–8, 18 July.

Spruyt, Bram, Gil Keppens and Filip Van Droogenbroeck, 'Who Supports Populism and What Attracts People to It?' *Political Research Quarterly*, Sage, 1–12, 2016, DOI: 10.1177/1065912916639138

'Unemployment Rate in India', Centre for Monitoring Indian Economy, https://unemploymentinindia.cmie.com/, 16 July 2020.

Upadhyay, Kavita. 2018. 'Inside the Ghost Villages of Uttarakhand', *Indian Express*, 24 June, https://indianexpress.com/article/india/uttarakhand-baluni-saina-bhootiya-abandoned-villages-migration-5230715/.

8

Unpredictable Lives and Livelihood with COVID-19

SANJEEV KUMAR MAHAJAN

The COVID-19 pandemic brought the world to a halt. Some parts are still in pause mode or are entering circuit-breaker lockdowns yet again. Many countries are trying different strategies to break the chain of the virus. The world is still struggling to collect specific statistics leading to the stabilisation of the situation. Numerous studies are being published continuously in reputed and peer-reviewed journals, which have left the scientific community befuddled. The inability to understand the virus as a result of its frequent mutations leaves the best minds in science unable to predict its onslaught in the future. Pharmaceutical companies and research organisations are struggling to develop a specific medical treatment for the virus. In India, as in other countries, math models to predict the exponential increase in the number of COVID-19 patients have failed for want of correct numbers. The numbers of deaths quoted by various state governments and the number of dead bodies (COVID deaths) brought to the crematoriums do not match. This is why no model seems to be working while predicting what will happen in the next few months.

The COVID crisis has posed a massive risk to people and the economy, except for a few small countries like New Zealand, Iceland, Tanzania, Fiji, Montenegro, Vatican City, Seychelles, Mauritius and Papua New Guinea. China, New Zealand and South Korea have managed to handle the pandemic relatively well. Amongst large countries, Australia and South Korea have withstood the impact of the coronavirus pandemic. Countries like India, Brazil and the US are struggling to keep the rising number of coronavirus-infected patients under control. The number of cases in India had crossed the 10.8-million mark as of 7 February 2021. The only solace for India is that the recovery rate is improving and is relatively better than many of the other developing countries. The current scenario has given a glimmer of hope that the world will win this pandemic war in the near future. For the time being, this myth was broken with the severe impact of the second wave in India, where, officially, 3.41 crore cases were registered and 4.53 lakh people died as on 21 October 2021. Scientists across the world have worked hard to create vaccines. However, it will take several years to inoculate every single person on the planet. Until then, unpredictability stares humanity in the face.

It is assumed that the pandemic has led to wide-reaching social and economic imbalances across the world. Moreover, this is the first such imbalance since the Great Depression of 1929. India's Gross Domestic Product (GDP) dropped to 5 per cent[1] in the first quarter of 2020, which was the lowest in the past six years. However, the situation became worse in the second quarter. International agencies have predicted a double-dip recession for India and the rest of the world. It looks like the world had underestimated the impact of the pandemic in its initial stages. This is primarily because 'there are two kinds of forecasters: those who don't know and those who don't know they don't know'.[2]

The pandemic has raised serious issues related to the strengths and weaknesses of governments at the national and state levels. The failure of governments to assess the unfolding of a crisis of this magnitude led to huge unpredictability, putting lives and livelihoods at peril. Predictability ignored in a period of non-predictability has affected lives and livelihood across the country. It is imperative to understand the political leadership's response to the unpredictability, especially during the ongoing pandemic. It is a gentle reminder to the world's economies that crisis management should top the agenda for risk management. International agencies such as the International Monetary Fund (IMF), the World Bank and the World Health Organization (WHO) have taken initiatives to provide funding to nations across the globe. Policymakers in different countries also need to come up with solutions for inclusive development to make the post-pandemic recovery sustainable.

Steps to Revive the Economy and Livelihoods

In India, the 2020–2021 and 2021–2022 budgets incorporated many policy initiatives to meet the challenges arising out of the pandemic. Along with the world, India faced challenges on both the supply and the demand sides.

The focus of the government now is on overall post-pandemic revival. Various segments such as healthcare, technology, education, unemployment, gender inequality and psychological health of the nation need an impetus for change.

Prescribing the Self-Reliance Pill

The COVID pandemic adversely impacted labour markets globally because of the strict lockdowns.[3] Although several nations have reopened, there are serious concerns about economic recovery. The pandemic has added fuel to the pre-existing global financial crisis.

India's GDP shrank by 23.9 per cent in the first quarter of the 2020–2021 fiscal year due to pandemic-induced disruptions, according to the data released by the Ministry of Statistics and Programme Implementation (MoSPI).[4] The chief economic adviser to the Government of India said in an interview that the GDP contracted by 7.3 per cent during the current financial year to ₹135.13 trillion in 2020–2021 from ₹145.69 trillion in 2019–2020. The Indian economy has suffered in both aspects—external and internal. External shock impacted export demand, tourism, foreign direct investment, etc. On the domestic front, measures to prevent the transmission of the contagious disease have resulted in steep reduction in the production of goods and services. Frequent lockdowns have adversely affected individuals as well as communities.

Figure 8.1: Economic Inferences of Restrictive Steps

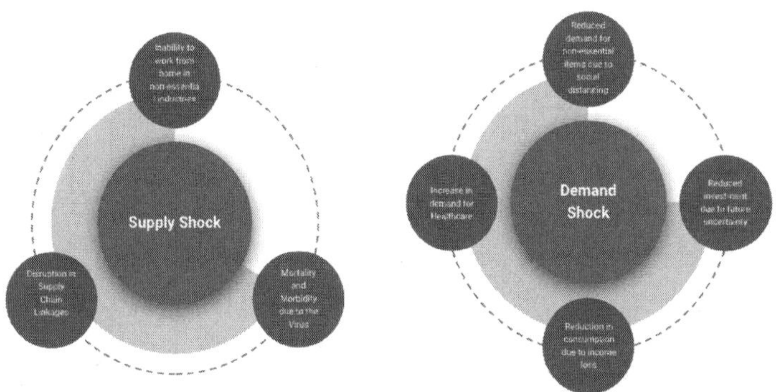

Source: Adapted from Estupinan, Xavier and Sharma, Mohit and Gupta, Sargam and Birla, Bharti (June 17 2020), 'Impact of COVID-19 Pandemic on Labor Supply and Gross Value Added in India'

The unanticipated global crisis and the repercussions of the pandemic have opened up new perspectives. It is now time to redefine and restructure policies and create new opportunities to put economic growth back on track. The declining GDP and increasing public debt have forced the political leadership to frame certain policies for the re-localisation of economic activities. The pandemic has prompted a disruption in employment and vulnerabilities in informal sectors. Enforcement of the lockdown resulted in inactivity in MSMEs.

The major initiatives that the GoI has taken to deal with the crisis are:

Focus on being *atmanirbhar* (self-reliant): The government initiated a Vocal for Local programme to develop India into an *atmanirbhar* or self-reliant economy to provide immediate and long-term relief to various business sectors. The five key focus areas of the Atmanirbhar Bharat initiative are: economy, infrastructure, systems (driven by technology), vibrant demography and demand.[5]

The Atmanirbhar Bharat initiative is meant to tackle five issues: Phase 1: Businesses, including MSMEs; Phase 2: Poor, including migrants and farmers; Phase 3: Agriculture; Phase 4: New horizons of growth; Phase 5: Government reforms and enablers.

Doling out economic packages: To revive the Indian economy, the government provided a special ₹20 lakh crore (equivalent to 10 per cent of the GDP) package on 13 May 2020. The focus was on making sustainable investments where the government and financial institutions were the stakeholders. This initiative was mostly meant to enhance and correct the supply chain disruptions. However, the release of money from the government to the states was a matter of concern. The government granted financial credit to different sectors, which are:

1. Concessionary credit to PM Kisan beneficiaries through Kisan Credit Cards (KCC).
2. Additional refinance support by National Bank for Agriculture and Rural Development (NABARD) for farmers.
3. Special credit facility to PM Street Vendor's AtmaNirbhar Nidhi beneficiaries, enabling easy access to working capital for street vendors.
4. Credit line under Emergency Credit Line Guarantee Scheme (ECLGS).
5. Extension of one-time restructuring of MSME accounts.
6. Extending the credit-linked subsidy scheme for housing for middle-income group till March 2021.[6]

The aim of the Atmanirbhar Bharat Abhiyan was that every individual is expected to create an opportunity for themselves for the betterment of the nation.

Goods and services tax: The legitimate transfer of compensation payments under the Goods and Services Tax (GST) implemented in 2017 came under severe stress post the pandemic. Under the GST arrangements, the states had let go of a portion of their rights regarding taxation as an alternative for the union government, relegating their share of revenue and indemnifying them from prospective revenue losses in the first five years.[7] During the pandemic, the clash between the union and the state governments escalated due to non-passing of the share to the states and non-payment under the financial cess. This aggravated the financial crisis in the states, resulting in fewer resources to invest in developmental activities. In many states, these activities came to a halt.

The GST collection has improved since October 2020 and is above ₹1 lakh crore currently. Besides, there has been a record collection of GST in April 2021. This proves that the economic activity is constantly improving. The amount collected under compensation cess is being shared regularly to businesses to ease their stress.

Building a More Robust Healthcare System

Tackling health problems has been a ceaseless struggle for everyone since eternity to lead a happy life. States, and not the centre, administer the healthcare system in India. The Union Ministry of Health and Family

Welfare executes various programmes related to the health and control of communicable diseases at the national level. It fosters traditional systems of medicine outside the Western allopathic ecosystems, such as Ayurveda, Siddha, Unani, Yoga, etc. It establishes standards and guidelines for the states for adoption.

Some of the steps taken to resolve healthcare issues and strengthen the healthcare infrastructure were:

Improving infrastructure: The UN Sustainable Development Goal (SDG) 3 says: 'Ensure healthy lives and promote well-being for all, at all ages.' India, committed to the UN SDGs, has been making efforts to formulate and amend policies for better delivery of health services. Healthcare infrastructure in India includes public, private and charitable care service providers. It has been observed that there are clusters of private care service providers in urban and semi-urban areas. It remained the duty of the government to develop healthcare infrastructure in rural areas, and the sector has shown tremendous improvement over the last few decades. Despite these improvements, the lacunae in the healthcare system came to the fore during the pandemic.

The rural–urban imbalance is also one of the factors that impeded access to the healthcare infrastructure. The primary, secondary and tertiary care institutions made the lives of the care seekers miserable. However, in the 2021–2022 budget, the government increased outlay for the health sector by 10 per cent. In its report, the Fifteenth Finance Commission recommended an increase of health spending to 2.5 per cent of GDP from the current 0.97 per cent of GDP.

Correcting the imbalance in the spread of COVID: It is an undisputed fact that India is a land of diversity, and this has been observed in the dissimilarity in the levels of infection, response and recovery from COVID in various states.[8] Ten states in India accounted for about 90 per cent of COVID infections in the first wave. In the second wave, the maximum number of cases came from the recently concluded poll-bound states and religious congregations held in March and April 2021. The pandemic has led to a change in priorities of the Indian healthcare system. Time-bound and limited resources have brought out the inefficiencies in the existing healthcare infrastructure. Healthcare experts and epidemiologists were unsure about the peak during the first wave of the pandemic in India and as doubtful or maybe even more during the second wave. India witnessed a fall in COVID cases towards the end of 2020 and at the beginning of 2021, which exploded in April 2021 again. As expected, India was not at all prepared for the second wave. This resulted in more pressure on the healthcare systems in the metros and the country's bigger cities.

India has limited healthcare infrastructure with only 713,986 beds, including 35,699 in intensive care units and 17,850 ventilators, according to a recent study by the Centre for Disease Dynamics, Economics and Policy (India) and Princeton University.[9] As per current estimates, the number of hospital beds has gone up to 1.9 million, ventilators to 48,000 and intensive care units to 95,000. The registered cases have surpassed the 26.7 million mark, and there are over 30 lakh active cases in India. There is a general perception among citizens that funds have not been allocated properly and that there is a lack of healthcare services in the country. The National Health Profile 2018 shows that India spends only 1 per cent of its GDP on healthcare infrastructure. In health infrastructure, India was ranked ninth by WHO among the ten countries in the region.[10]

Lowest ranking in health infrastructure: It is clear from the report of National Health Profile 2019 that 12 states ranked below the national average on bed availability (the national figure was 0.55 beds per 1000 population). There is an acute shortage of hospital beds in India. Policymakers are at a loss regarding finding solutions for critical care patients and in providing ventilator support.[11] The state governments have been trying hard to keep hospitalisations low by encouraging people to exhibit COVID-appropriate behaviour and mandatorily wear masks in all public places. This statement holds value in the context of the second wave. It has been observed that hospital infrastructure nearly crumbled in April and May 2021. There was a lack of availability of beds, intensive care units as well as ventilators. On top of this, many hospitals faced an acute shortage of oxygen and medicines.

In 2020, India had zero production of PPE and critical care equipment such as ventilators. Over time, these capacities were built. The union, state and district level governments have motivated and urged private, public and non-profit agencies to provide essential goods and services by using the latest information and technology mechanisms.[12] In the absence of sufficient hospital equipment, medicines and oxygen, the GoI accepted international medical aid.

Meanwhile, routine healthcare programmes with specific reference to immunisation, care for the elderly, pregnant women and children have taken a back seat during the pandemic. Many reports suggest that the Outpatient Department (OPD) in several hospitals are closed for the public. The situation does not seem to be improving in the near future. Many scientists are now predicting the third wave that might hit hard India in the latter part of 2021. The prediction is that children will bear the brunt of the third wave. Paediatrics-related infrastructure has to be upgraded at the earliest if the scientists' warning comes true. Though the governments at the central and state levels have learnt lessons from the outcome of the second wave and have been preparing for it, it would not be wise to let their guards down till the pandemic is over.

Meandering Through a Psychological Crisis

Such a long-drawn pandemic has a massive impact on both the physical and the mental health of people. Even though the COVID crisis focuses essentially on the physical health of people, it is soon becoming a psychological one for which measures must be taken.[13]

Anxiety and stress weigh down many sections of the population, especially frontline health workers, the elderly, women and children. Most of us are scared of physical isolation, infection, dying or fear of losing a family member, which adversely impacts our mental health. This apart, millions of individuals have started facing economic instability because of losing their jobs and reducing incomes.

There has also been a change in lifestyle as we aren't travelling as much as before. New challenges have emerged in the form of working from home (WFH) and homeschooling children, social restrictions such as avoiding contact with family members, friends and colleagues. The fear of the pandemic circulating through electronic and social media platforms added to people's anxiety. A United Nations (UN) report and policy guidance on COVID acknowledged that the pandemic had gravely impacted the mental health and happiness of individuals.

On 18 March 2020, the WHO issued guidelines to support different target groups' mental health and psychological well-being, such as healthcare workers, leaders managing health facilities, children, the elderly and those living in isolation. Actions need to be a part of the national policy regarding the response to COVID. The WHO firmly believed that a concerted effort from parents, teachers and the government was necessary to help children cope with the crisis and thrive in the post-pandemic world.[14]

Focus on Keeping Domestic Violence in Check

It was observed in many studies that women face systematic disabilities. They face deprivation, power domination and inequity in many sociopolitical structures.[15] Cases of violence against the vulnerable segments of the population markedly rose due to many reasons after the pandemic.

Several domestic violence incidents were recorded in the first four months of the lockdown in India, as seen in the table below.

Table 8.1

Type of Violence	*Never told anyone*	*Told someone*	*Sought help from a source*
Physical	79.5	9.6	11.6
Sexual	80.6	9.5	9.8
Physical and Sexual	61.3	9.9	28.8

Source: https://www.thehindu.com/data/data-domestic-violence-complaints-at-a-10-year-high-during-covid-19-lockdown/article31885001.ece

The majority of the victims said they would never share their experiences with others. Very few dared to seek help from relevant authorities. Domestic violence has been a complex issue plaguing society, and data suggests that the number of incidents rose dramatically post the pandemic. This observation was recently validated in a report by the department-related Parliamentary Standing Committee on Home Affairs. The committee observed that an increase in domestic violence cases took place because of disruption in economic activities, work from home and families remaining together for more time during the lockdowns.[16] Realising the gravity of the situation, UN Secretary-General Antonio Guterres appealed to all governments via social media to prioritise women's safety during the pandemic.

The only way to deal with domestic violence is to stigmatise the behaviour of the guilty rather than to offer counselling support from time to time. Another way is to launch aggressive nationwide campaigns to kindle awareness in society.

Dealing with Wrath of Redundancies

Unemployment and its impact on the people's psyche was another massive problem that the lockdown brought along, and a large number of businesses had to shut shop. In states like Maharashtra and Delhi, statistics show that unemployment drastically increased since the exodus of migrant labourers in March 2020.[17]

The pandemic hit the global economy hard. It has been a massive blow to the Indian economy too, especially with the GDP on the decline since the first quarter of the 2019–2020 financial year. Global rating agencies have projected 0.8 per cent GDP for the FY 2020–2021.

Table 4.2 Statistical Profiles - Unemployment in India

Month	*Unemployment Rate (%)*		
	India	*Urban*	*Rural*
Jan 2021	6.53	8.08	5.83
Dec 2020	9.06	8.84	9.15
Nov 2020	6.50	7.07	6.24
Oct 2020	7.02	7.18	6.95
Sep 2020	6.68	8.45	5.88
Aug 2020	8.35	9.83	7.65
Jul 2020	7.40	9.37	6.51
Jun 2020	10.18	11.68	9.49

May 2020	21.73	23.14	21.11
Apr 2020	23.52	24.95	22.89
Mar 2020	8.75	9.41	8.44
Feb 2020	7.76	8.65	7.34

Source: https://unemploymentinindia.cmie.com/, retrieved on 7 February 2021

Unemployment in India spiked during April and May 2020. The overall unemployment was highest (at 23.52 per cent) in April 2020, but since then, the numbers have started improving. If India wants to ramp up its economic growth, there must be diligent strategising.

The pandemic has severely hit the following four sectors:

Micro, Small and Medium Enterprises (MSMEs): The MSMEs, engaged in manufacturing and export activities, are the bedrock of the Indian economy. During the lockdown, this sector came to a grinding halt, which otherwise contributes over 30 per cent of the GDP. During the first quarter of FY 2020–2021, the sector contracted by 39 per cent. It is also important to note that the sector is one of the top job creators for the country.

Tourism: The pandemic has dealt a brutal blow to the tourism, hospitality and aviation sectors. A KPMG report predicted that the Indian tourism and hospitality sectors would lose more than 3.8 crore jobs.[18] According to the data released by MoSPI for the first quarter, trade, hotel and other services shrunk by 47 per cent. Experts believe that this sector will be the last one to resume activities. Looking at the gravity of the problem, the Ministry of Tourism has asked the premier institution

National Council of Applied Economic Research to study the impact of this pandemic and economic losses for households engaged in the tourism sector in January 2021.

Real estate: Construction activities came to a standstill following the lockdown. Although they have resumed partially, key projects are still on hold. These two sectors were key employment generators for migrant workers.

Mining: India produces over 85 minerals. Minerals and ores are the essential ingredients of many primary industries. The mining sector growth slipped 23 per cent due to the pandemic.

Ethics and COVID-19

According to WHO, the virus causing COVID-19 is SARS-CoV-2.[19] The priority of every government is to combat the scourge of the pandemic and build the economy. But corruption has flourished during these troubling times. Although anti-corruption measures and accountability systems are in place, various sections of society have raised their voice against alleged misuse of resources. A former chief minister of Karnataka has alleged that a ₹2,200 crore scam occurred in the purchase of COVID-related equipment.[20] Similar accusations have been made in the purchase of dead-body bags, bedsheets and thermometers in Maharashtra by the leader of the opposition.[21]

Governmental agencies have to ensure that public funds are being used judiciously. These are testing times for the government and the ideal time to build people's trust in its institutions. Policymakers must ensure equity, independence, interdependence and unanimity.

Not Taking Eyes off the Development Goals

The biggest question staring the government in the face is how to revive the economy, especially now in the wake of the immense second surge. The government had initiated the move to become *atmanirbhar* as COVID presented a unique opportunity to bridge the gap in the economy through well-defined policies to improve public infrastructure.

The pandemic has made a severe dent in the overall progress of the UN Sustainable Development Goals (SDGs). To achieve SDGs within the stipulated time, a country needs to invest smartly in its healthcare system and infrastructure (in a digital and environmentally conscious way) to improve lives and livelihood.

The Indian government has taken extraordinary policy measures to enhance the usage of and dependence on digital technology.

The story of India's digital journey has been one of transformation and inclusion. The digital revolution has led to transparency and inclusive growth (productivity and efficiency). In India, social assistance has been provided to vulnerable sections of society, such as migrant workers and farmers, via direct digital and online transfers to beneficiary accounts. In India's lockdown period, from 24 March 2020 to 17 April 2020, the direct benefit system (DBT) was used as the main instrument to transfer ₹36,659 crore to the bank account of 16.01 crore beneficiaries. This was possible only because the Pradhan Mantri Jan Dhan Yojana was launched in 2014 to provide universal access to the banking sector.

The pandemic has also disrupted the education sector and has left millions of students in the lurch. Students of all ages, especially in low- and middle-income countries, face inadequate access to quality education. To safeguard students, policymakers need to seriously think about investments in the education sector and how best to improve the distance learning capacity.

Recently, Prime Minister Narendra Modi,[22] for the first time, talked about the centre–state *bhagidari* (participation) on his blog on LinkedIn. The GoI is committed to raise enough resources for public welfare. He further highlighted that the Atmanirbhar Bharat Abhiyan has started showing positive results. The focus remains on improving the ease of living, especially for the poor, the vulnerable and the middle class. This is only possible through fiscal sustainability. India can only meet challenges by having faith in the federal polity and moving ahead in the right spirit of centre–state *bhagidari*.

9

Education for Education

VINAY SHARMA

On 7 March 2020, I was going through my planner. It was the festival of Holi in India. 11 March, I had to reach back IIT, Roorkee. 12 March had to be a busy day, and many tasks including classes and meetings had to be accommodated and prepared. Mid-semester exams were over and the plan for the next part was fixed. It had to be revamped and restructured, conforming to the requirements of the coming times, including some project-level commitments. March also calls for the financial closing. Financial utilisation certificates and reports had to be put in for funding organisations. Intermediary project completion reports were to be submitted. Besides, some conferences were coming up in June and July, so preparations had to be done and papers had to be finalised. The upcoming schedule was packed and 100-odd tasks had to be completed within the next 4–5 months. Everything was to be reworked, so I flipped through the pages of the planner and started shifting my commitments at the right places on the relevant dates. Just to mention that I use traditional planners and jot down a to-do list.

On 11 March, I boarded a night train from Lucknow to Roorkee and reached the next morning. Meanwhile, news was pouring in that COVID-19 has knocked the doors of our country. The authorities were active and identifying suspected carriers and the temperature of travellers was being monitored at airports. This did not sound alarming enough, though rest of the world was already battling the virus since December 2019. Several questions popped in my mind. Was I not aware of the facts? Did it not come to my mind even once that I should feel concerned? Actually not. Daniel Kahneman in *Thinking Fast and Slow* has explained reasons of such a response and there are other researchers who have explained 'human behaviour and response'. Does it mean that COVID-19 was not actually so silent and it is the people who have not been behaving the way they should?

COVID-19 Already Stepped In

There were news items claiming that it is already in Mumbai or Delhi, and that IIT Roorkee campus, where I work, would not be so immune to the virus. On 15 March, everyone was told that things would go out of hand, and the next day we decided not to invite students on mid-semester break back to the campus. Subsequently, I called my research scholars and advised them to go back home. 'Let the situation come back to normal in 2–3 weeks,' I told them. Why did we expect the pandemic to weaken within a few weeks? Were we confident of our resources? For the first time ever the entire campus was deserted. A few walkers were seen wearing a mask although reluctantly. There was an air of general disbelief about the lockdown and wearing of masks almost as if humanity was being challenged. The lockdown week which started with a call of a day went into the presumption that things might not be so out of hand and still my planner was alive and I was shifting all the 100 plus tasks to some other dates in the near future. By 19 March this exercise had to be repeated once again, when on the same night the Prime Minister of India declared a *janta* curfew on 22 March and addressed the nation on 24 March declaring a nationwide lockdown starting midnight of 24–25 March 2020.

This forced vacation directed my thoughts to things which faintly existed at the back of my mind, such as exercise, yoga, walking, a weight reduction plan, reading books, watching films and documentaries and talking to family and friend; It felt like an opportunity.

Still Predicting

So, I had planned that a fortnight later I would be working over time to catch up lost time. Two weeks later the planner which had been a guiding force became absolutely irrelevant. All the dates became irrelevant. Online discussions and meetings began with an intent to find a solution to the situation.

Predictive Modelling Was Not Helping

The entire education system which had been directed towards predicting and forecasting was trying to find answers. Post 19 months, we still are doing that and acknowledging the fact that a radical change must be thought of, but we all know that 'it is not us who start with a clean slate, complexities write themselves off at their own discretion'.

Stop predicting, said COVID-19 in 2020 and has been loudly saying that in 2021 as well.

'Stop predicting' is the catchphrase, COVID-19 has taught the education world. This should not be taken as something wrong or detrimental. Students, scholars, teachers and all the beneficiaries of education always wanted a change. Institutions wanted to re-emphasise the value of knowledge against tangible output orientation and results. Everyone was feeling entrapped. COVID-19 has compelled the world of education to focus on dissemination. Institutions and teachers are worried about not being able to reach out to students.

Evaluation without examination is the test of the system itself. Most importantly, the changes are here to stay. The task of change is evident as a testimony. A striking fact being that not only was a quick adaptation witnessed but several innovative methods were being developed and experimented upon. In March 2020, all the students were preparing for exams and the teachers were busy with planning for exams, evaluation and the next sessions. Colleges and universities were discussing the routine and expansion. Increasing the number of students and courses has been a parameter of growth, which was being pursued strongly. Everyone, even distantly related to the subject, was talking about the National Education Policy 2020, appreciating the futuristic direction, flexible approach and a desirable trajectory.

Abrupt Stop and Silence

Suddenly everything stopped. Institutions, schools, colleges and coaching centres were deserted. Everyone was in for a homebound surprise vacation. 'Let's use the time' was the phrase going around. See you after 2–3 weeks, was the adieu. Uncertainty had crept in. Let's get in touch with the students, was the message. Ideas started flowing and modes of communication became pertinent and information and communication technology was ready to extend the much-needed support.

A Model Evolved

Practices of large, established, prosperous and technology-enabled institutions became the benchmark. Surprisingly it did not require a lot of investment. Education became mobile, and an era of the mobile-based education emerged. There have been discussions around this and advertisements suggesting the mobile phone as a mode of disseminating education, but no one knew that this would come so soon, without much persuasion and would be adopted almost instantaneously. Parents who were reluctant in handing over electronic devices to their children started sparing their own mobile phones and started purchasing new hardware. Newer methodologies which would be more effective were improvised and meta-marketing of several associated devices came to the fore. S-Pens, writing pads and several other recording devices became prominent. Newer software, connecting platforms and networks, along with ever-increasing bandwidth and storage space, became the point of concern for several large organisations in keeping with the desire of the customers and users. These modes alone could save the situation, and perhaps nothing would be lost. Though the flow of technological adaptation has been magically fast but accessibility has always been a very big question. Connectivity as well as purchasing power to deal with reliable hardware supporting interaction is necessary for attending sessions but is beyond the reach of millions. This has been depressing for children and many resorted to drastic steps. We were not ready for the need of such magnitude, though we have always been acknowledging that communication and communication technology should be accessible to all. An important aspect which has been witnessed is that the country not only has the acumen but the will and resources to bring up the solution for the problems which are emerging in relation to this unprecedented change. Please refer to the link where Himanshu Shekhar Mishra, one of the co-authors of this book, reports on what the government is doing proactively (https://www.ndtv.com/india-news/use-satellite-tv-to-beam-classes-for-poor-students-amid-covid-parliamentary-panel-to-centre-2469128.)

Let's Go Back for a While

For decades, we wanted a much broader dissemination of education. The concept of open universities, content for everyone, access to libraries and breaking free from any restriction was meticulously pursued. It came up as an open and alternative education. The objective was transformation through access, and the goal was to raise the level of skills. We all know this story. We all have been a witness to the spread of education, the associated struggle for infrastructure, teachers, functional literacy and employability, etc. An incremental innovation to support this struggle came up in the form of e-content, later becoming e-courses.

Online and Offline

The term online assumed greater significance in this scenario. Though it is used for several purposes, it became prominent largely because of online education. Education was never called offline. May 2020 converted the complete education dissemination system into an online system. You must have heard people saying something like 'it must be going online at your end... yes, and is it the same at your end as well? Yes, it is'. Getting reassured that everyone is on the same page reduces the anxiety of losing something, and institutions transited to fulfill the requirements of their curriculum. Postponement of lab work, delaying of exams and other such actions were taken, but we still were predicting the end to the crisis. At the same time, we were planning a rejuvenation of the system after restoration of some kind of normalcy. Some newspapers and channels are reporting that the reopening of the institutions is being planned for July, whereas discussion on forthcoming waves of COVID-19 is also on.

A system which has always been largely closed ended with a specific structure, where attending classes, taking exams and qualifying have been the static features leading to planning years in advance. The question is of establishing the linear progression of a child's education, from the entrance exam he would appear for to the course he would be eligible for and the kind of institution he would enroll in have been an interwoven thought process. Industries like 'coaching' centres grew at a very large scale due to this structure. It may take a newer shape as the framework is realigned and its pace may revert to its original structure, but the students in transit are left perplexed. Why couldn't we be flexible? Why is reaching to the institution amongst institutions always an uphill task? Why is education in the form of knowledge not flowing unhindered as rivers do?

Have We Really Learnt Our Lessons?

We had lessons to learn then and probably many lessons to be learnt now as well. The second wave came in or it can be said that another spurt of spread of the virus was seen and devastatingly experienced, which compelled another transition with writing off of the steps and processes. Exams got shelved. Algorithms, simulations, videos, virtual labs and many other innovative steps replaced activities that were essentially physical in nature. Many institutions and stakeholders who did not have access to sophisticated tools started evaluating completion of syllabi and courses without practice. The 'net gain' philosophically took over 'net loss'.

A Painful Transition

This transition carried the weight of anguish and pain. When things were opening up, our predictive understanding deceptively motivated us to imagine pre-COVID normalcy after fulfilling some protocols. Everything was going right, we were moving ahead, students were back to their colleges, children started joining schools and we were about to declare the virus as 'gone' when it suddenly exploded. Many experts had warned, but everyone was anxious to get over it. COVID-19 took over everything devastatingly as COVID-20.

There was silence everywhere. Fear took over. This time the victims were young adults, who got infected enmasse. Mass isolation and mass return to homes came up as a frightful exercise.

Unchanged Desire of the Outcomes

Despite it all, the desire of outcome of education never changed. An astonishing fact was that educational institutions successfully positioned education as a product associated with a price-based benefit analysis and estimation. The result is parents not depositing the fee and many college students demanding their fee deposits back.

The college and professional education students are expecting 100 per cent placements, which is not wrong, but it presents a paradox that is related to the economic progression not being conducive. Though it has been observed that the students are willing to divert from the levels of profiles that they desire, a reluctant mild compromise on the levels of the pay packages has also been observed though not in consonance with the economic changes. Institutions and organisations went for salary cuts, layoffs and employers extended their dates of joining and even diverted their offers along with rescinding their jobs.

A Confusing, Disheartening State for All

For someone who was waiting for a struggle to end post his education and also for someone who was struggling to get education, the situation has posed a darkness of sorts. Why is there such a confusion? Is it true that the education earned or education delivered till now would not be effective or would not be comparatively effective because of the change of environment and process of dissemination? Is it also true that if the courses would not finish in time, it would be creating a detrimental effect throughout the life of the student? Is it true again that if the courses would not result in the next step, say placements or jobs for the college students, the whole exercise would completely go waste? If the answers to all these questions are even partially yes, then something with reference to the delivery and dissemination of education from conception to the end must not have been done right. We all know that the prime purpose of education is to gain knowledge, implying that if this has been fulfilled then the core objective has been achieved.

But by this stage of the discussion and revisiting the last 24 months from November 2019 to November 2021, one feels lost and perplexed. The fundamental thought being that the situation should revert to as it was.

An Introspection

Is this an opportunity? A blow? A barrier? A transition or something else?

Let's Stop Predicting the Professional Outcomes

All the textbooks and courses define their learning objectives. These objectives mention the outcomes. Those outcomes up till a few months back have been specific to the learning of a student yielding an understanding for an application. Outcomes and objectives gradually got structured into being professionally oriented, so much so that students started looking into the specific tangible gains out of every learning.

All the subjects, starting from the preparatory class to the end of the course, have been meticulously interwoven into a sequential learning as if a specific road reaching to a particular job. That makes sense if the conceived picture of the future gets a shape as imagined. For example, a strong agrarian economy pursuing micro-enterprise and nurturing a dream of self-reliance gets diverted to the services, and by the time one realises, a large pool of talent carrying its knowledge goes away to serve in different countries.

COVID-19, while instigating economic problems, has volumes of lessons for 'educating us in delivering education'. One realises that the sequential orientation and the plan of education we had in mind must have been right, but it requires knowledge as the major outcome which is utilised for different purposes during such a time but also instigate innovation. Knowledge is the key for us to understand our fundamental duty as human beings, to participate with our means in fighting such wars and atleast keep ourselves safe so as to support the warriors. Knowledge is the key to not fall into an entrapment of profit as the parameter. It is a key to be innovative, to run the economy as well as for diverting the skills and orientation of human resources towards the productive processes. There could be a question: Can education develop such a 'capability' so as to instil multifaceted human resource which may change its course overnight? The answer is yes, and it is not rhetorical because there are examples if we look around.

Education must empower either to expect the unexpected and to be ready or to change the course as and when required. The crux of the matter is that why can't learning be such that the outcomes may be decided by the choice of the students or their future course itself. Literature tells us that we had learning systems and universities which taught the students to live in consonance with the present while caring for the future and reminiscing the fact that humans have come for humans and would live for humans.

Another question is: Did a pandemic have to tell us about how we should have pursued education? Did education itself have to learn from the incident?

Not, actually, because education is the giver and has the capacity to unearth gems and hone them till they sparkle.

But who does that? Educationists do that at large. Did they go wrong somewhere?

Educationists did not predict the outcomes of the education other than wisdom.

The role of educationists and education had been to facilitate this whole narrative of living, and somehow when humans started getting confident about controlling things, they realised that they should direct all the learning towards profits and benefits. They started utilising each other as a resource, and the whole education system directed its attention to train people rather than to make them learn. It was structurally decided which kind of people would do what in their lives and how they would do that. The outcomes were measured in terms of the role they would play and the relative compensation they would get. These were the only two measurement criteria which have been existing for the past 4–5 decades. The world invariably kept on following that; education and educationists started focusing on the benchmark model and kept incrementally complimenting it, whenever it was necessary. An important question to an educated person now is: 'What salary do you get?' and 'Where do you work?'

Does it have something to do with COVID-19? You should decide, I suggest. Readers who have faced the pandemic know where I stand when I write this, and readers who know about this devastation through spoken or written references would also feel connected to this argument.

National Education Policy 2020 also desires a change and has been released at a time when this is required most. Once again, a report by Himanshu Shekhar Mishra on the potential of NEP 2020 will help you in visualising the changes India foresees in the entire education system (https://www.ndtv.com/india-news/national-education-policy-nep-pm-narendra-modi-says-government-intervention-influence-should-be-minimal-2291495.)

The question though is that do we have the people and gurus to take it further? Do we have people who are ready to switchover careers with a radical orientation and deep understanding? How would this be achieved?

The answer is simple. We have to bring the people who can facilitate this process without inhibition and listen to them and follow them. Identification of people who are reflective is not difficult at all. We just have to look for them. How? In today's data analytics days we just have to follow lectures, videos and research of such people and teach the teachers.

What should be done?

The role of an educationist has always been related to an initiative to specifically revisit everything and to imagine, not only about what should be the outcome but also

a) in terms of content and pedagogy,
b) in terms of interest,
c) in terms of attracting students towards the meaning of education, not as an avenue of getting jobs but to learn.

It is the creativity of academicians at the individual level which would turn things towards an everlasting meaningful course. Have you read *Tuesdays with Morrie*? It is a beautiful read and you would understand my intent of mentioning 'creativity' of academicians.

How and Why?
Revisiting Objectives, Processes and Outcomes

It is interesting when we talk about revisiting objectives and processes and outcomes because revisiting not only means retrospective perspective of everything but also means that we have to create a new picture of correlation amongst the elements. It may mean that we should think in terms of linking up natural elements with each other as nature does. The success of acting upon the lessons lies in the fact that 'education must plan to eliminate greed as an outcome of the processes.' Does it sound rhetorical? It also implies reducing weightage given to rankings and ratings. Will it reduce constructive competitiveness? Will it reduce efficiency? Am I sounding like I am taking the complete system back to the ancient times? The answers are not complex at all. Please go back to your planners and simply write: I intent to learn something. A lesson for life from life. A lesson of science from life. A lesson of art from life. The next day, just write the lesson you have learnt. After a few years you would be handing over the crux of your life to someone or the world at large in one single sentence or a few keywords.

Let me explain this with a short story. While introspecting during my student days, I realised that I may not have learnt much from my parents and teachers whom I admired and who have done so much in their lives. Fortunately, during my early career days, I got a chance to stay with my parents, who practiced medicine by profession and served the state government health department. I have been a witness to their hard work and their truthfulness to the profession and oath. Once I asked my mother to tell me in a few words about what she did throughout her life? Her simple answer in a few words contained the story of a long journey of penance. She said, 'I served thousands and thousands of patients without discrimination and performed hundreds of thousands of surgeries without failure by the grace of God.' I asked my father the same question one day and the answer was similar: service to mankind by the grace of the Almighty. They always said that we also raised our children. Does one require any further explanation on the criteria of output of one's education?

The Discussion May Go On

It would be prudent for me not to mention what 'we do' or 'we should do' but 'what we can do' because many years later students might still face a question on 'what would they be doing?'. Someone might refer to the clues. Discussions on COVID would remain there forever, accompanied by the turning points it brought in. I imagine an inquisitive mind going through this book, reaching to this section and probably agreeing to not being anxious on tangible achievements education might bring to him, but to think about nurturing a purpose.

So let's see what can we do? Let me start with the perspective of parents and teachers of children. It would be redundant to mention discussions about what everyone wishes for a child to become. That is not wrong because if it would not be so then many children would not have been trained for what they did for the whole of their lives. The question is of the content of the training and education imparted to them. What was required to propel a child for her entire life to find a purpose and nurture it? Was it the languages she learnt? The mother tongue, the spoken language, the language of science, maths, computer programming, music and several others. A language is the reason for life. It is not an exaggeration if you talk to a soldier and ask him how he interprets his life and he would proudly mention his oath and duty. So where and how did it divert? Was it related to the interpretation of languages or a cross-language thought process which made us multilingual with jumbled thoughts?

Speaking of languages, I remember the names of my teachers who taught me words and their context.

After working with several organisations, one fine morning I decided to become an academician. Though it is like any other story of struggle and then gaining satisfaction and fulfilment, it restrengthens the value of education when you really wish to search for a sense of purpose. In 2008, when the world was reeling under an economic recession and my students were worried about their careers and future, I was in a situation to narrate my experience of finding a sense of purpose and could motivate many to strive for excellence and dedication through their knowledge. One fine day, I was writing an abstract of a paper and suddenly realised that the art of precis writing which was taught to me by my teacher Shri Vidya Bhushan Chaturvediji came handy. After around 30 years I called him when I realised the beauty of the gift he gave me. Within a few seconds he recognised me from the other side. I could sense the warmth and satisfaction of his smile after he learnt that I had became an academician. I tried to think up a few words that I will someday pass on to someone as a legacy I inherited from my teachers.

What Has COVID-19 Got to Do with All This?

A growing organism looking for life made us carriers and unleashed itself in no time, leaving us wondering what kind of a problem it is or the kind of problems it will bring. We know it is a virus and that it understands survival with multiplication. Thousands of research papers were published within a year's span, leave aside articles and debates, compelling us not only to wonder about the magnitude of the problem but also to think that fighting this war requires an integrated problem-identification methodology and integration of languages we work with which actually could not be effectively pursued because of the functional compartmentalisation we designed.

More than 18 months later, we are wondering how to look at it. Is it a biological problem? Yes, it is. But can the solution be brought about only through biological research? No, it must be coupled with an understanding of the supply chain, distribution systems, economic aspects along with the structures of cities and remoteness of villages. The production of essentials has to be done; agriculture has to go on, though the workforce has to be confined. Above all, communicating with the masses to take precautions, about steps to be taken in case of infection, to work but with care and most of all about where we stand. When would it go if at all it would? Why it may come back and why not? What kind of similar problems are ahead of us? And the biggest question which must be raised, discussed and answered by the teachers, researchers and academicians is: 'How should people be thinking about living their lives from now on? Should they change their dreams? Should we be redefining our aspirations, the meanings of the terms that drive us and the benchmarks and measurement criteria we had been following and pursuing?

Who would guide us on such complex, interlinked and urgent questions?

Education has guided us and will guide us through. It is just that we must embrace it as it should have been, which is for the purpose of gaining knowledge and living our lives. Here in the end, sharing my anguish with everyone. I refrain from denouncing 'forecasting' altogether but do emphasise that we must stop predicting! Let's refrain from saying that 'something will happen'. Let's learn to say that 'we should respond and live, whatever happens'. Remember education never ends; it lives forever.

Conclusion

Towards a Post-COVID-19 World

VINAY SHARMA
RABINDRANATH BHATTACHARYYA
SANJEEV KUMAR MAHAJAN
HIMANSHU SHEKHAR MISHRA

With more than 4 lakh new cases added on a single day on 8 May 2021,[1] India's official total tally of coronavirus infections reached more than 3 crore at the end of June 2021, making it the third country after the US and Brazil to have crossed 3.97 lakh deaths due to COVID.[2] It is an evolving situation as the virus is constantly mutating, and once again no one is able to predict to what extent the infection will spread or when the third wave and then, if any, fourth wave will come. This reminded us about everything that took place in the third week of March 2020. The lockdown had not been declared yet. People were still going to their workplaces without masks, but there were obvious loud whispers that some kind of stringent measures were going to be imposed to fight an unknown enemy called the coronavirus.

Hand sanitisers were almost sold out, surgical masks were not available and people were scared to step out of their homes or to meet even the closest of friends in person. People were also in a dilemma whether or not to allow domestic help and if their services were to be suspended, and for how long. Subsequently, the lockdown was declared from the midnight of 25 March when the number of confirmed COVID-infected patients stood at 564 (*The Hindu*, 24 March 2020). At that point, there were no SOPs to treat COVID patients. Doctors had very little knowledge of how to take care of such patients, and there were no separate hospitals for them. There was also a social stigma attached to such patients. While all this was happening, the police and law enforcement agencies were focused on implementing the lockdown in the country. By the second week of February 2021, the COVID curve had somewhat flattened and new cases came down to less than 10,000 a day in India. Once again, people began predicting what the future would hold.

Human behaviour is usually oriented to two basic objectives: comprehending a situation and then predicting the outcome while relying on that comprehension. However, a major danger of such predictive modelling is the acceptance of bias and variance that leads to the peril of overfitting, something that happened with the COVID situation as well. In 2021, tourism started to thrive again. Live cricket started to entertain all of us. Religious festivals such as Holi were celebrated without paying much heed to the pandemic protocols. Election rallies and processions were attended by lakhs of maskless people. On 15 March 2021, The *Economic Times* reported an '80% drop in sale of masks and sanitisers' over the lockdown period.

But at the end of March 2021, the second wave hit the country in an aggressive manner. The Kumbh Mela was suspended halfway at the end of April 2021, and on

4 May 2021, the Indian Premier League (IPL) matches were suspended indefinitely after multiple players and support staff tested positive for COVID.[3] Quoting one health economist, *BBC News* reported on 26 May 2021 regarding India: 'The seven-day rolling average of new reported cases during the wave peaked at 392,000 and has been on a steady decline ever since for the past two weeks.'[4] Throughout the chapters, it was seen how the first wave and then the second wave of the pandemic hit various walks of life. People were looking for answers to so many questions: Where is the end of this pandemic? How many waves will there be? Will there be light after this darkness? Will lives be back to normal again? Keeping in mind all these questions, the authors have attempted to explore the lessons of COVID without predicting any end to this pandemic.

The second wave was distinct in terms of the oxygen crisis and the violation of COVID protocol during the last rites of patients. Despite this, there is a marked similarity in the situation between the second wave of 2021 and the first wave of 2020—and that is unpreparedness. All countries, including India, in 2021 knew what kind of a health infrastructure, medical and medicinal support coronavirus-infected patients required. In 2020, there was a lack of diagnostic kits which India had to import from neighbouring countries. This was no more the case in 2021 with India manufacturing the diagnostic kits. Doctors had the SOPs in place to treat patients. Insurance companies, too, had COVID covers in place. People also learnt the ways and means to deal with the pandemic and help one another. But then, the policymakers were confident in their prediction that India had won the war against COVID. That mistake brought with it a lackadaisical attitude in planning for an aggressive vaccination programme throughout the country or developing oxygen plants, which needed little investment, for medical treatment. The nation survived the crisis, but at the cost of a huge number of precious lives.

Lessons Learnt

The pandemic is a hard taskmaster. It taught many lessons that will not be forgotten for generations to come. Both the policymakers as well as civil society learnt how to react/respond/live with an unpredictable situation. We will highlight some of these great lessons while concluding this book.

The first lesson that we have learnt is the need for new legal provisions to deal with the pandemic. One of the examples is the amendment of the century-old Epidemic Diseases Act, 1897, to The Epidemic Diseases (Amendment) Act, 2020 (Gazette of India, notification on 29 September 2020). The powers of the central government to conduct inspection of any ship, bus, train, goods vehicle, vessel or aircraft as well as the detention of any person trying to leave a port during an epidemic was specified. Protection for healthcare personnel and damage to property were also specified in the Act. This has further established a new pandemic protocol at the national level that has put in place a viable policy framework for regulating vaccine production, deployment and nationwide vaccine rollout identifying the beneficiaries. Such a new legislative response, after developing a national consensus among political parties, state governments and union territories, is critically needed to undertake new institutional steps. These legal provisions will help strengthen India's medical and healthcare facilities. The new law should also help reform its crisis communication protocol and strengthen the existing public health communication systems on the ground. The new law must outline the blueprint for an outbreak risk communication plan to fight such public health exigencies in the future.

The second major lesson from the pandemic is that the development paradigm on the linear growth model, which focuses on consumerism, may hit social lives hard during a pandemic. The COVID crisis has been a lesson in the basics of well-being in a way that may sustain the lives of the people. The pandemic taught us to look at a larger cost analysis and acknowledge the fact that all the people, be it the leadership or the general masses, should think of prosperity and happiness of the world in a collective manner. It has taught us that development starts with a sustainable interconnection between human beings and nature. It has taught us that catering to linear consumption-based growth may not serve the purpose of development. Policymakers should think about how to avoid disasters and how to maximise peace, happiness and sustainability rather than how to optimise it. It hinges on a fundamental system of well-being which says that there should be access for everyone to food, health, education, decent livelihood, gender equality, clean water and sanitation, a pure environment and so on. The pandemic has taught us that the sky is one and so is the sea for all those living on this planet. So clean water, pollution-free air and an ecological equilibrium should be appreciated and protected. They must not be sacrificed at the altar of development. That way, there is also a need to rationalise consumption-based infrastructure currently in use.

On a different plane, this crisis has also reflected the inherent challenges for the marginalised population as well as the community as a whole. A crisis of this proportion calls for us to revisit how we perceive life, what it takes to be resilient and to work together as a society. The pandemic has shown us all that we do not require much for living a reasonably decent life. It has demonstrated that when consumerism reduces, development gets a new meaning by recalibrating demand and supply. The pandemic, in a sense then, has made a positive impact on human well-being by pushing self-aggrandisement to the backburner by giving environment a new lease of life and by encouraging innovation. It has showed that the contingency plan as a ready referral may lose its relevance at any point of time, but that does not mean that negativity has won. Rather, it leads to a certain flexibility and ingenuity.

The third major lesson of this pandemic is the necessity of keeping the social memory alive with perfect storage of historical data. Each country has grappled with biological disasters at some time or the other on a small or large scale. The present pandemic, however, shook the world because we did not learn any lessons from the previous ones, especially from the Spanish flu of 1918. Enough data was not available about the previous pandemics. The agencies need to refurbish themselves to meet the challenges arising out of the current pandemic. Awareness campaigns regarding the ill-effects of the virus and the pandemic need a lot of focus from the government, private organisations, non-profit civil society organisations, research institutions as well as from local authorities. Citizens must also learn to deal with this, so that lives and livelihoods remain protected as much as possible. All will not be the same in a post-COVID world. We will have many changes in our lifestyles as well as community rituals and celebrations. Perhaps the mask will become the new normal for a long time to come. So, the various aspects of such a world-shattering pandemic should be a part of academic curriculums at various stages.

Post-COVID Challenges

We do not know for how long we will have to live with COVID. The third wave or even the fourth wave may occur, and the economy depends heavily on how long India will have to battle the pandemic. Such disasters have a debilitating impact on the forces of production as they cripple trade and economic processes, disrupt supply chains and create a demand–supply mismatch. This makes the economic recovery process in the post-disaster phase difficult, complex and prolonged. Millions of displaced migrant workers are still struggling to cope with the pandemic.

Considering the devastating impact of the pandemic across important sectors of the Indian economy and the currently looming uncertainty, the vision of economic revival trajectory remains a difficult and complex one. Different assessments have been made by Indian and global agencies about the nature and timeline of economic revival in the post-pandemic world. India's Economic Survey 2020–2021, tabled in Parliament on 29 January 2021, argued that 'the economy would take two years to reach and go past the pre-pandemic level'. The survey is optimistic about the prospects of an economic revival in FY2021–22.[5] It categorically asserts: 'After an estimated 7.7 percent pandemic-driven contraction in 2020–21, India's real GDP is projected to record a growth of 11.0 percent in 2021–22 and nominal GDP by 15.4 per cent.' The finance ministry's Department of Economic Affairs, in its Monthly Economic Review (MER) report for February 2021, cautioned:

> A major downside risk to growth continues to be the pandemic induced morbidity and fatality that has elevated health stimulus as a key macroeconomic lever for India's continued economic recovery. Rapid production and deployment of COVID-19 vaccination will be critical to taking forward the health stimulus deep into FY 22.[6]

In the MER report released in May 2021, it has been observed that

> In India, the pace of contagion in the second wave has been alarming, stretching the health infrastructure in terms of the capacity to handle a surge of this size and speed. A decline in seven days moving average of new cases since 8 May 2021 and seven days moving average of active cases since 13th May 2021 marked the attainment of the peak of the second wave—almost 4 times the peak in the first wave. Given the ferocity of the second wave, the spread of infection in rural areas has also been rapid.'[7]

As per the report, it is significant to reach herd immunity as early as possible for the purpose of economic recovery. The report mentions the meaning of herd immunity as the immunity or less susceptibility to infection of 80 per cent of the population.

The challenges India face today go far beyond the severe contraction of its economy. Herd immunity through vaccination is now the basic challenge. The pandemic has posed unprecedented governance-related challenges since the first case of COVID infection was reported in Kerala on 10 January 2020. It would be imperative to promulgate a new law to address the broader challenges India has faced and strengthen its legislative framework to combat future pandemics. Moreover, the government, central or state, should take the onus of providing basic infrastructure of the well-being of citizens like free vaccines, oxygen during medical emergency or enough crematoriums so that the dignity of corpses is not violated. Realisation of an ideal state or Ram Rajya in the Gandhian concept—ensuring equal rights for a prince and a pauper alike, reflecting true democracy—may be a long-term idea. But striving towards that ideal will always be a great drill for policymakers towards self-discipline and community well-being.

In the End

India ignored the larger lessons of the Spanish flu of 1918. It cannot afford to ignore the lessons that the COVID crisis has taught us. If one does not learn lessons from one's mistakes, it is highly likely that the same mistakes will be committed again. The world has faced a disaster of this magnitude after a century. The mitigation of the biological disaster requires a multi-dimensional approach. Authorities at the central and state levels need to be realistic, make enlightened policy decisions and facilitate adequate arrangements to invest in controlling and overcoming the challenges posed by the pandemic.

Finally, there is a need to highlight the positive gains as well. Many lives, known as well as unknown, were lost—a scar on the community that will require long time to heal. Nevertheless, there were many unsung heroes who fought day and night to provide people relief and the courage to come out of their sufferings. There was a huge network of collective actions that put humanity first. Society, in an innovative manner, has developed many new normal habits like working from home, shopping on e-commerce platforms or flexible education through the internet. Parents got opportunities to spend time with their children, which wasn't always possible due to everyone's busy schedule. The lockdown, including stopping of flights, domestic as well as international, had a positive impact on the environment, including noise pollution, greenhouse gas emissions and air pollution. The pandemic caught us unawares and taught us many harsh lessons. We now have SOPs for managing a pandemic. But do we have an SOP for managing life that may keep such a pandemic away in the future? As Bob Dylan said, 'The answer is blowing in the wind.'

Appendix

Legal Provisions for Disaster Management in India

Constitutional Provisions

There are different provisions in the Constitution of India that cover dimensions concomitant to development and livelihood and the protection and development of the environment and natural resources. These constitutional provisions are[1] given below:

Article 21 of the Indian constitution states that no person shall be deprived of his life or personal liberty according to the procedure established by the law. The commutation of this article means that the government has to make tenable efforts to be resilient in the wake of disasters. That is, emphasising creating adequate infrastructure to reduce risks.

Article 38 says the state shall strive to promote the welfare of the people by securing and protecting as effectively as possible a social order in which justice, social, economic and political, shall inform all the institutions of national life.

Article 48A states that the state shall endeavour to protect and improve the environment and safeguard the country's forests and wildlife.

Article 51A(g) talks about the duty of every citizen of India to protect and improve the natural environment, including forests, lakes, rivers and wildlife. Every citizen should have empathy for the living organism.

Apart from these constitutional provisions, the state is also responsible under the doctrine of *parens patriea*.[2] The doctrine of *parens patriae* makes it obligatory on the part of the state or the supreme authority to safeguard persons with disability. Although the doctrine was supposedly opposite to King, the judiciary made it mandatory for the states to impart relief to disaster-affected people. The concerned ministries, designated as nodal agencies, have been responsible for dealing with the disaster. Many laws have been enacted or amended by the union and the state governments according to the needs of the time.

Disaster Management Plan

The initiatives taken by the GoI for disaster management include setting up various committees and passing certain relevant Acts.

A High Powered Committee was set up in 1999 under the chairmanship of J.C. Pant to devise an inclusive, systematised and integrated approach for the first time since Independence in 1947. This committee made some cogent plans for disaster management at the national, state and administrative levels.[3]

In 2002, the government set up the National Committee on Disaster Management, with the prime minister as its chairman, after the earthquake in Gujarat. It included representatives from political parties at the national and state levels. The committee was responsible for making disaster risk mitigation and resilience management plans.

This chapter focuses on just those Acts that specifically deal with the current COVID-19 pandemic. We will look into the Disaster Management Act of 2005 and the Epidemic Disease Act of 1897.

The basic objective of the Disaster Management Act of 2005[4] was to dispense for the constructive management of disasters. After the implementation of this Act, the focus shifted towards disaster mitigation, prevention and preparedness. The Act was also known as the mother Act to deal with disasters (natural or man-made). Disaster management under the Act referred to a sustained and unified process of planning, organising, coordinating and implementing measures that are imperative for[5]:

1. Prevention of danger or threat of any disaster.
2. Mitigation or reduction of risk of any disaster or its severity or consequences.
3. Capacity-building.
4. Preparedness to deal with any disaster.
5. Prompt response to any threatening disaster situation or disaster.
6. Assessing the severity or magnitude of effects of any disaster.
7. Evacuation, rescue and relief.
8. Rehabilitation and reconstruction.

The Disaster Management Act of 2005 has eleven chapters and seventy-nine sections extending over entire India. The purpose of this Act is to provide an effective governance of disasters and their associated consequences. The Act provides for a three-tier structural system to manage disasters (National Disaster Management Authority, State Disaster

Management Authority at the state level and District Disaster Management Authority at the local/district level) to meet these challenges. Under the Act, the central government's responsibility is to establish the National Disaster Response Fund and National Disaster Mitigation Fund to deal with any emergency disaster situations arising in the country.

The legal implications arising from these offences and penalties have been elaborated in Chapter X (Section 51–60) of the Disaster Management Act of 2005. It also brings forth civil and criminal liabilities for the violators not adhering to the Act's provisions.

The Epidemic Disease Act of 1897 came into existence to overcome the bubonic plague epidemic during the colonial era. The bubonic plague broke out in the province of Bombay in the last decade of the 19th century. The purpose of this Act was to confer special powers to the local authorities to implement requisite measures to control the epidemic effectively. Its most important feature was that it was one of the shortest legislations of India. It contains only four sections. Interestingly, this Act did not apply to the former state of Jammu and Kashmir (now divided into two union territories). However, a separate Epidemic Act of 1977 was enacted by Jammu and Kashmir.

Section 2 of the Epidemic Disease Act empowers the union and state governments to promulgate special actions that can be taken to repress the spread of diseases. Section 3 deals with the provisions of penalties for the violation of regulations, similar to Section 188 of the Indian Penal Code, that is, disobedience of order enforced by a public servant. Lastly, Section 4 describes the provisions concerning legal protection provided to public servants while implementing the Act.

Limitations of the Epidemic Disease Act, 1897

Although this Act was implemented essentially for controlling the bubonic plague, it remained inactive since Independence. It was invoked recently during the coronavirus pandemic but failed to live up to the expectations in the rapidly changing scenario. The physical attacks on doctors and other healthcare workers and damage to public and private properties led to a revaluation of the Act's provisions to address its ability to tackle such attacks and acts of social exclusion. The GoI brought out an ordinance, keeping in mind the urgency of the situation.

The government passed the Epidemic Diseases (Amendment) Ordinance on 1 April 2020 by amending the Epidemic Disease Act, 1897. The main aim of this ordinance was to protect healthcare professionals and provide a secure environment to them as they perform their duties. Both Houses of Parliament passed the legislation. This legislation provides for up to five years in jail for those attacking doctors and healthcare workers during the pandemic.

The Objective of the Post-Pandemic Ordinance

The Epidemic Diseases (Amendment) Ordinance was brought in 2020 primarily to protect doctors and healthcare workers who were constantly coming under attack from hapless patients and their families, and also to prevent any damage to property during a pandemic.[6] The salient features of the ordinance are:

1. Violence under the ordinance: It focuses on zero tolerance for violence and harassment of and any physical injury to healthcare service professionals and damage to property.
2. Penal provisions: This has been introduced to deal with offences that have been classified into three categories, and there is also mention of penalties to be imposed.
3. Investigation of offences: The investigating officer should be no less than the rank of inspector. The investigation must be completed within 30 days, and the trial has to be completed in one year.
4. Healthcare professionals: A healthcare professional refers to any empowered person who can take measures to prevent and control the disease. Doctors, nurses, paramedical workers and community health workers are named as healthcare professionals. State governments have been empowered to include any such category which it deems fit to be incorporated by issuance of notifications in official gazettes.

Twinning Disaster Management with Sustainable Development

Disaster management covers all facets of planning, coordination and implementation of action to prevent or minimise the effect of a disaster. This can only be possible if the nation has an effective and proactive disaster management framework in place. It is expected that disaster management activities have to blend with developmental activities. India and Yokohama Strategy of the UN International Decade of Natural Disaster Reduction follow the integration of disaster risk reduction strategy. It is appropriate to say that disaster risk reduction is the core strategy focusing on sustainable development.

The three authorities that were entrusted with ensuring implementation and execution of the Disaster Management Act of 2005 were the National Disaster Management Authority (NDMA), State Disaster Management Authority (SDMA) and District Disaster Management Authority (DDMA).

According to Section 3 of the Disaster Management Act, the prime minister chairs the NDMA. The vision of this group is 'to build a safer and disaster resilient India by a holistic, proactive, technology-driven and sustainable strategy that involves all stakeholders and fosters a culture of prevention, preparedness and mitigation'.[7] Section 6 of the Act states that it is the responsibility of the NDMA to lay down policies, plans and guidelines for effective disaster management to ensure an effective response to the disaster. There is also a provision to constitute an advisory committee comprising experts in areas of disaster management. The NDMA has created a National Executive Committee and sub-committees to assist in its performance as defined in the Act.

A National Disaster Management Plan was also put in place, whereby regulations were laid down for public agencies to handle all aspects of the disaster management cycle. These were in keeping with the provisions of the Disaster Management Act of 2005 and guidelines of the National Policy on Disaster Management (NPDM), 2009. The central vision of NPDM is to: 'Make India disaster resilient across all sectors to achieve substantial and inclusive disaster risk reduction by building local capacities, starting with the poor and decreasing the loss of lives, livelihoods and assets in different forms, including economic, physical, social, cultural and environmental, significantly while enhancing the ability to cope with disasters at all levels.'[8]

The NDMP, in a sense, has five main pillars.[9]

1. Aligning with the DM Act 2005 and the NPDM 2009.
2. Dynamic engagement to achieve the global goals according to the agreements to which India is a signatory—Sendai Framework for DRR, Sustainable Development Goals (SDGs) and Conference of Pares (COP21) Paris Agreement on Climate Change.
3. Prime Minister's Ten-Point Agenda for DRR, articulating contemporary national priorities.
4. Social inclusion as a pervasive principle.
5. Making DRR a dominant attribute.

The NDPM has recognised the need to minimise the responsibility framework by following an integrated approach. This will help ensure proper involvement of governmental and non-governmental agencies, the private sector and the local communities at large. It will also provide a clear role for quick mobilisation of resources by all the stakeholders.

Let's now move on to see how SDMA and DDMA can help. According to Section 14 of the Disaster Management Act of 2005, each state government shall set up an SDMA, which will comprise a chairperson and other members (not more than nine). SDMA aims to lay down policies and plans and take measures for prevention, mitigation and preparedness to deal with disaster situations in states with a thrust on capacity-building.

According to Section 25, Chapter IV of the Act, each state government shall set up a DDMA in every district. The deputy commissioner will head the DDMA with a co-chairperson, an elected representative of the local authority. The DDMA will act as the planning, coordinating and implementing agency, according to the guidelines laid down by the NDMA and SDMA. The role of the NDMA, SDMA and DDMA are to prepare for disasters, mitigation and prevention.

Here's how disaster risk management and mitigation shall work.

Figure A.1: Process of Disaster Risk Management and Mitigation

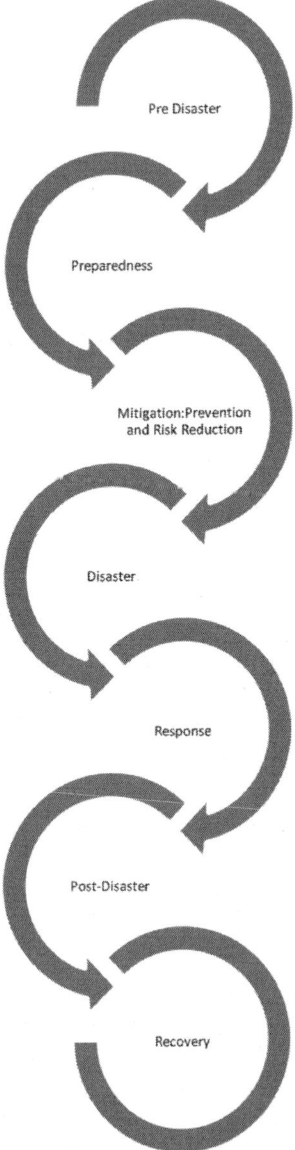

Source: https://ndma.gov.in/images/policyplan/dmplan/ndmp-2019.pdf. Page 2

ABBREVIATIONS

AI	Artificial Intelligence
BMC	Brihanmumbai Municipal Corporation
BARC	Broadcast Audience Research Council
CDC	Centers for Disease Control and Prevention
CMIE	Centre for Monitoring Indian Economy
CII	Confederation of Indian Industry
CSR	Corporate Social Responsibility
DBT	Direct Benefit System
DDMA	District Disaster Management Authority
EC	Election Commission
ECLGS	Emergency Credit Line Guarantee Scheme
EEMA	Events and Entertainment Management Association
FAO	Food and Agricultural Organization
FCI	Food Corporation of India
FAQ	Frequently Asked Questions
GAAP	Generally Accepted Accounting Principles
GHI	Global Hunger Index
GST	Goods and Services Tax
GoI	Government of India

GDP	Gross Domestic Product
GoM	Group of Ministers
ICMR	Indian Council of Medical Research
IMD	India Meteorological Department
IOS	Industrial Outlook Survey
IMF	International Monetary Fund
IOM	International Organization for Migration
KCC	Kisan Credit Cards
ML	Machine Learning
MGNREGA	Mahatma Gandhi National Rural Employment Guarantee Act
MGNREGS	Mahatma Gandhi National Rural Employment Guarantee Scheme
MP	Member of Parliament
MSME	Micro, Small and Medium Enterprises
MoSPI	Ministry of Statistics and Programme Implementation
MER	Monthly Economic Review
NABARD	National Bank for Agriculture and Rural Development
NCR	National Capital Region
NCW	The National Commission for Women
NDMJ	National Dalit Movement for Justice
NDMA	National Disaster Management Authority
NDRF	National Disaster Relief Fund
NFSA	National Food Security Act
NPDM	National Policy on Disaster Management
NSS	National Sample Survey
ONORC	One Nation One Ration Card

OPD	Outpatient Department
PPE	Personal Protection Equipment
PMGKY	Pradhan Mantri Garib Kalyan Yojana
PMGKAY	Pradhan Matri Garib Kalyan Ann Yojana
PCI	Press Council of India
PIB	Press Information Bureau
PM CARES	Prime Minister's Citizen Assistance and Relief in Emergency Situations
PMO	Prime Minister's Office
PDS	Public Distribution System
SOP	Standard Operating Procedures
SDMA	State Disaster Management Authority
SDRF	State Disaster Relief Fund
SDG	Sustainable Development Goal
UN	United Nations
WFH	Work from Home
WHO	World Health Organization

NOTES

CHAPTER 1 EXPECT EVERYTHING—IT'S WAR

1 Office of RK Singh, Minister of State (IC) Power and New & Renewable Energy, 30 June 2021. https://twitter.com/OfficeOfRKSingh/status/1410232232837476362?s=08

2 Express News Service. 2021. 'Last words of nursing officer who helped countless patients at Delhi's Lok Nayak hospital: "Mujhe bacha lo"', *Indian Express*, 1 May, https://indianexpress.com/article/cities/delhi/last-words-of-nursing-officer-who-helped-countless-patients-at-delhis-lok-nayak-hospital-delhi-covid-7298189/.

3 Anuradha Mascarenhas. 2021. '747 doctors died of Covid-19 in India: IMA', *Indian Express*, 17 April, https://indianexpress.com/article/cities/pune/747-doctors-died-of-covid-19-in-india-ima-7277087/.

4 PTI. 2021. 'Over 30,000 children orphaned, lost a parent or abandoned due to COVID-19, NCPCR tells SC', *Economic Times*, 7 June, https://economictimes.indiatimes.com/news/india/over-30000-children-orphaned-lost-a-parent-or-abandoned-due-to-covid-19-ncpcr-tells-sc/articleshow/83308281.cms.

5 Srishti Jha. 2021. 'SC Directs Centre To Frame Guidelines For Compensation To Families Of COVID-19 Deceased', *Republic World.com*, 30 June, https://www.republicworld.com/india-news/law-and-order/sc-directs-centre-to-frame-guidelines-for-compensation-to-families-of-covid-19-deceased.html.

6 'Ramjayya', https://www.mkgandhi.org/momgandhi/chap67.htm.

7 Shri Ramcharitmanas by Goswami Tulsidasji with Hindi Text and English Translations (Gorakhpur: Gita Press, 2019).

8 PIB. 2020. 'English Rendering of Prime Minister Shri Narendra Modi's Address to the Nation on 12.5.2020', 12 May, https://www.pib.gov.in/PressReleasePage.aspx?PRID=1623418.
9 Governor's Statement, Reserve Bank of India, 17 April 2020, https://rbidocs.rbi.org.in/rdocs/Content/PDFs/GOVERNORSTATEMENTF22E618703AE48A4B2F6E-C4A8003F88D.PDF

CHAPTER 2 A REALITY CHECK

1 Kimberly Hickok. 2020. 'What Is a Pandemic?', *Live Science*, 13 March, https://www.livescience.com/pandemic.html.
2 Agencies. 2020. 'India declares Covid-19 a "Notified Disaster"', *Economic Times*, 14 March, https://economictimes.indiatimes.com/news/politics-and-nation/india-declares-covid-19-a-notified-disaster/articleshow/74631611.cms.
3 'UNISDR Terminology on Disaster Risk Reduction', United Nations International Strategy for Disaster Reduction, 2009, https://www.unisdr.org/files/7817_UNISDRTerminologyEnglish.pdf.
4 Amartya Bag. 2009. 'Indian Federalism: Examining the Debate', SSRN, 5 November, https://papers.ssrn.com/sol3/papers.cfm?abstract_id=1500315.
5 Amartya Bag. 2009. 'Indian Federalism: Examining the Debate.' Retrieved from: https://papers.ssrn.com/sol3/papers.cfm?abstract_id=1500315 on 10 July 2020
6 Amartya Bag. 2015. 'From Disorganised Effort to Organised Polarisation of Corporate Social Responsibility in India.' In *Asian Governance: Paradoxes of Development*. Edited by Akrbaruddin Ahmad and Suman Sharma. Bangladesh: Policy Research Centre, B.D. Foundation, 152.
7 General Circular No.15/2020, F. No. CSR-01/4/2020-CSR-MCA, 10 April 2020. Ministry of Corporate Affairs. Government of India. New Delhi.

CHAPTER 4 PANDEMIC NARRATIVE AND THE MINDSET OF CIVIL SOCIETY

1 Amitabh Sinha. 2021. '3 lakh Covid-19 deaths in India: How far is the second wave peak?', *Indian Express*, 1 June, https://

indianexpress.com/article/explained/india-covid-situation-coronavirus-deaths-how-far-is-peak-7328929/

2 Prabhash K. Dutta. 2021. 'Bodies Found Floating in Ganga. Can Rivers Spread Covid-19?' *India Today*, 12 May, https://www.indiatoday.in/coronavirus-outbreak/story/bodies-found-floating-in-ganga-rivers-spread-covid-19-1801740-2021-05-12. This was also reported in other media. Kumar, Sudhir. 2021. 'Over 80 bodies found in Ganga in UP, Bihar', *Hindustan Times*, 12 May, https://www.hindustantimes.com/india-news/over-80-bodies-found-in-ganga-in-up-bihar-101620759387610.html.

3 Abhishek Mishra. 2021. 'Prayagraj: Burial of Bodies in Sand Old Custom but Never Saw So Many, Say Locals', *India Today*, 24 May, https://www.indiatoday.in/india/story/uttar-pradesh-prayagraj-ganga-river-bank-dead-bodies-buried-sand-1806086-2021-05-24. This was again also reported in other news organisations. ANI. 2021. 'Bodies Found Buried in Sand on Banks of Ganga in UP's Prayagraj', *Hindustan Times*, 16 May, https://www.hindustantimes.com/india-news/bodies-found-buried-in-sand-on-banks-of-ganga-in-up-s-prayagraj-101621162366236.html.

4 India Today Web Desk. 2021. 'Oxygen Emergency Worsens Covid Crisis: How to Fix It?' *India Today*, 22 April, https://www.indiatoday.in/coronavirus-outbreak/story/covid-crisis-oxygen-cylinder-shortage-solution-apollo-hospitals-dr-sangita-reddy-1794020-2021-04-22; The Hindu Net Desk. 2021. 'Coronavirus Updates',*The Hindu*, 21 April, https://www.thehindu.com/news/national/coronavirus-live-april-21-2021-updates/article34372726.ece;Yadav, J.P. 2021. 'Covid-19: Modi Silent on Oxygen Crisis', *Telegraph*, 26 April, https://www.telegraphindia.com/india/covid-19-pm-modi-mum-on-oxygen-crisis/cid/1813678.

5 Thucydides. 2009. *The Peloponnesian War, Book II.* Translation by Martin Hammond, Oxford World's Classic.NewYork: Oxford University Press, 173.

6 Thucydides. 2009. Ibid., 173.

7 Alfred W. Crosby. 2003. *America's Forgotten Pandemic—The Influenza of 1918*. UK: Cambridge University Press.

8 Gina Kolata. 2005. *Flu—The Story of the Great Influenza Pandemic of 1918 and the Search for the Virus That Caused It.* New York: Touchstone.

9 Worldometer, 28 June 2021. https://www.worldometers.info/coronavirus/

10 'Global COVID-19 Death Toll More than Double Official Estimates – IHME', Reuters, 6 May 2021, https://www.reuters.com/business/healthcare-pharmaceuticals/global-covid-19-death-toll-more-than-double-official-estimates-ihme-2021-05-06/.

11 Lazaro Gamio and James Glanz. 2021. 'Just How Big Could India's True Covid Toll Be?' *New York Times*, 25 May, https://www.nytimes.com/interactive/2021/05/25/world/asia/india-covid-death-estimates.html.

12 Jamie Mullick. 2021. '1 in 5 Fatalities Old: Pandemic Toll Rises as States Reconcile Numbers', *Hindustan Times*, 13 June, https://www.hindustantimes.com/india-news/1-in-5-fatalities-old-pandemic-toll-rises-as-states-reconcile-numbers-101623523653390.html.

13 Special correspondent. 2021. 'Coronavirus | 18-44 Age Group May Get COVID-19 Jabs Only through Private Facilities', *The Hindu*, 26 April, https://www.thehindu.com/news/national/coronavirus-18-44-age-group-may-get-covid-19-jabs-only-through-private-facilities/article34407310.ece.

14 Krishnadas Rajagopal. 2021. 'Supreme Court queries on equity, pricing nudge change in vaccine policy', *The Hindu*, 7 June, https://www.thehindu.com/news/national/supreme-court-queries-on-equity-pricing-nudge-change-in-vaccine-policy/article34755905.ece.

15 G. Harvey 'On the Original, Contagion, and Frequency of Consumptions.' In Gideon Harvey, *Morbus Anglicus*. London: Nathaniel Brook, 1666: 2–14, as cited in Morens, David M., Gregory K. Folkers and Anthony S. Fauci, 2009. 'What is a pandemic?' *The Journal of Infectious Diseases, Oxford Academic*, Oct 1; 200(7):1018–1021.

16 Retrieved from: https://www.who.int/csr/disease/swineflu/frequently_asked_questions/pandemic/en/

17 David M. Morens et.al. 2009, pp. 1018–1021.

18 Crosby. 2003. *America's Forgotten Pandemic—The Influenza of 1918*, page 102.

19 ———. page 105.

20 ———. page 109.

21 'Guidelines Regarding Covid', National Health Mission, 12 March 2020, http://nrhmhp.gov.in/sites/default/files/files/Dissemination%20of%20mask.pdf.

22 'SOP on preventive measures to contain spread of COVID-19 in offices', Ministry of Health and Family Welfare, https://www.mohfw.gov.in/pdf/1SoPstobefollowedinOffices.pdf.

23 Express News Service. 2020. 'Kerala Government Makes Facemask, Social Distancing Mandatory for One Year', *New Indian Express*, 5 July, https://www.newindianexpress.com/states/kerala/2020/jul/05/kerala-government-makes-facemask-social-distancing-mandatory-for-one-year-2165771.html.

24 ANI. 2020. 'Jharkhand to Impose ₹1 Lakh Penalty, 2-Year Jail Term for Violating Covid-19 Norms', *Hindustan Times*, 23 July, https://www.hindustantimes.com/ranchi/jharkhand-to-impose-rs-1-lakh-penalty-2-year-jail-term-for-violating-covid-19-norms/story-JC7ttUFGgqLYWduO9rYTVO.html.

25 PTI. 2020. 'Not Wearing Mask? Work as Volunteer in Gwalior Hospitals, Police Check-posts', *Deccan Herald*, 6 July, https://www.deccanherald.com/national/north-and-central/not-wearing-mask-work-as-volunteer-in-gwalior-hospitals-police-check-posts-857673.html.

26 Jerryl Banait Vs. Union of India & Anr. 2020. https://main.sci.gov.in/supremecourt/2020/10795/10795_2020_0_5_21591_Order_08-Apr-2020.pdf

27 Joe Wallen. 2020. '"They Said They Would Murder Me': Pandemic Sees Rise in Attacks against India's Lowest Caste"', *Telegraph*, 29 June, https://www.telegraph.co.uk/global-health/science-and-disease/said-would-murder-pandemic-sees-rise-attacks-against-indias/; Divya Trivedi.2020. 'Report Exposes Increase in Atrocities against Dalits; Former CJI KG Balakrishnan Calls for Better Law Enforcement', *Frontline*, 15 September,https://www.im4change.org/latest-news-updates/report-exposes-increase-in-atrocities-against-

dalits-former-cji-kg-balakrishnan-calls-for-better-law-enforcement-divya-trivedi.html.

28 Thucydides. 2009, p 99.

29 Firstpost. 30 September 2020. https://www.firstpost.com/india/unlock-5-0-guidelines-announced-cinema-halls-can-reopen-with-50-capacity-states-to-decide-on-resumption-of-schools-from-15-oct-8867301.html.

30 Lakshmi Govindrajan Javeri. *First Post*, 25 June 2020.

31 Gaurav Laghate. 2020. 'India Records Highest TV Consumption in a Week with Total Time Spent of 1.27 Trillion Minutes', *Economic Times*, 25 June 2020, https://economictimes.indiatimes.com/industry/media/entertainment/covid-19-impact-tv-consumption-reached-a-historic-high-of-1-2-trillion-minutes-in-a-week/articleshow/74951009.cms?from=mdr on 8 August 2020.

32 Shyamala Venkatachalam. 2020. 'Coronavirus Crisis: Why Television Industry is Bleeding Despite Record Consumption', *Business Today*, 5 May, https://www.businesstoday.in/opinion/columns/coronavirus-outbreak-covid-19-television-industry-bleeding-despite-record-consumption/story/402868.html.

33 PTI. 2021. '70 Lakh Participated In Kumbh Mela Held Amid Covid Surge', NDTV, 1 May, https://www.ndtv.com/india-news/70-lakh-participated-in-kumbh-mela-amid-covid-19-surge-2425654; PTI. 2021. 'Kumbh Mela Ends, 70 Lakh Participated in "Scaled Down" Event Held amid Covid Surge', *India Today*, 1 May, https://www.indiatoday.in/india/story/kumbh-mela-ends-70-lakh-participated-scaled-down-covid-surge-1796833-2021-05-01.

34 Thucydides. 2009, pp. 96, 173.

35 Crosby. 2003, page 25.

36 ———. page 37.

37 Miranda Bryant. 2021. 'Third Wave of Covid "Definitely under Way" in UK, Says Expert', *Guardian*, 19 June, https://www.theguardian.com/world/2021/jun/19/third-wave-of-covid-definitely-under-way-in-uk-says-expert.

38 Riya Baibhawi. 2021. 'COVID-19: Europe Battered With 3rd Wave, France Tops Infection List As UK Gears For Unlock', *Republic World*, 4 June, https://www.republicworld.com/

world-news/uk-news/covid-19-europe-battered-with-3rd-wave-france-tops-infection-list-as-uk-gears-for-unlock.html.

39 Madhuparna Das. 2020. 'Funeral of Bengal's COVID-19 Patient Triggers Protest, 16 People Arrested', *Print*, 24 March, https://theprint.in/india/funeral-of-bengals-covid-19-patient-triggers-protest-16-people-arrested/387071/.

40 PTI. 2021. 'As Death Toll Spirals, Corpses Wait in 20-Hour Queues for Last Rites at Delhi Crematoriums', *DT Next*, 27 April,https://www.dtnext.in/News/TopNews/2021/04/27190250/1290500/As-death-toll-spirals-corpses-wait-in-20hour-queues-.vpf.

41 Kangana Sachdeva. 2021. 'Dead Bodies Piled Up on Pavement outside a Crematorium in Ghaziabad Allegedly Due to Shortage of Space Inside', *Times Now*, 16 April, https://twitter.com/timesnow/status/1382977043575410688?lang=en; Mishra, Stuti. 2021. 'India Coronavirus: Bodies Piling Up at Delhi Crematoriums and Human Remains "Burned next to Pavement"', *Independent*, 19 April, https://www.independent.co.uk/asia/india/india-covid-deaths-delhi-crematorium-b1833776.html.

42 The Print, 16 April 2021. https://theprint.in/india/dead-bodies-all-over-lucknow-funerals-tell-a-story-starkly-different-from-up-govts-claims/640741/

43 Yagnesh Bharat Mehta. 2021. 'Five bodies Cremated on Single Pyre in Surat', *Times of India*, 16 April, https://timesofindia.indiatimes.com/city/surat/five-bodies-cremated-on-single-pyre-in-surat/articleshow/82094745.cms,

44 Ashna Butani. 2021. 'Final Rites on Pavement outside Crematorium, Ghaziabad Administration Says Part of Facility', *Indian Express*, 19 April, https://indianexpress.com/article/cities/delhi/ghaziabad-crematorium-footpath-covid-patient-bodies-7280587/.

45 Geeta Pandey. 2021. 'Covid-19: India's Holiest River is Swollen with Bodies', BBC, Delhi, 19 May, https://www.bbc.com/news/world-asia-india-57154564.

46 https://www.prsindia.org/sessiontrack

47 'Budget Session of Parliament Adjourns Sine Die; A Total of 18 Bills Passed by Both the Houses of Parliament; The Session Saw a Productivity of Approx. 114% in LokSabha and 90% in

Rajya Sabha', PIB *Delhi*, 25 March 2021, https://pib.gov.in/PressReleaseIframePage.aspx?PRID=1707544

48 'Allahabad High Court Issues Notice to State Election Commission on 135 Teachers' Death on Poll Duty', *Tribune*, 28 April 2021, https://www.tribuneindia.com/news/nation/allahabad-high-court-issues-notice-to-state-election-commission-on-135-teachers-death-on-poll-duty-245372,

49 'Congress Brings Up Pre-Poll Promise of Free Vaccination in Bihar; Urges Centre Not to "Burden" States to Procure Vaccine', *Hindustan Times*, 14 May 2021, https://www.hindustantimes.com/india-news/congress-brings-up-pre-poll-promise-of-free-vaccination-in-bihar-urges-centre-not-to-burden-states-to-procure-vaccines-101620987482109.html.

CHAPTER 5 COVID-19 AND THE CHALLENGE OF CRISIS COMMUNICATION

1 Prime Minister's Office. 2020. 'Text of Prime Minister's Address to the Nation on Combating COVID-19', PIB, 19 March, https://www.pib.gov.in/PressReleasePage.aspx?PRID=1607254.

2 NDTV, 3 March 2020, https://ndtv.in/videos/impact-of-corona-virus-increses-in-india-saleing-of-sanitizer-increased-542194.

3 Debanish Achom. 2020. 'Price of 200 ML Hand Sanitizer Can't Be More than ₹100: Government', NDTV, 20 March, https://www.ndtv.com/india-news/coronavirus-update-price-of-200-ml-hand-sanitizer-cant-be-more-than-rs-100-says-government-2198205

4 Prime Minister's Office. 2020. 'Text of Prime Minister's Address to the Nation on Combating COVID-19', PIB, 19 March, https://www.pib.gov.in/PressReleasePage.aspx?PRID=1607254.

5 Ibid.

6 Prime Minister's Office. 2020. 'PM Interacts with Electronic Media'. 23 March, https://www.pib.gov.in/PressReleasePage.aspx?PRID=1607684.

7 Prime Minister's Office. 2020. 'Text of PM's Address to the Nation on Vital Aspects Relating to the Menace of COVID-19', PIB, 24 March.

8 PTI. 2020. 'No Panic Buying Please: PM Says Essentials, Medicines To Be Available', NDTV, 24 March, https://www.ndtv.com/india-news/coornavirus-lockdown-prime-minister-narendra-modi-says-essentials-medicines-to-be-available-2200118.

9 Nilanjana Bhowmick. 2020. '"They Treat Us Like Stray Dogs': Migrant Workers Flee India's Cities', *National Geographic*, 27 May, https://www.nationalgeographic.com/history/2020/05/they-treat-us-like-stray-dogs-migrant-workers-flee-india-cities/; Soutik Biswas. 'Coronavirus: India's Pandemic Lockdown Turns into a Human Tragedy', BBC World, 30 March, https://www.bbc.com/news/world-asia-india-52086274.

10 Prime Minister's Office. 2020. 'Principal Secretary to the Prime Minister Chairs a High-level Meeting on Coronavirus outbreak', PIB, 25 January, https://www.pib.gov.in/PressReleasePage.aspx?PRID=1600552.

11 Amit Shah Rally, 29 January 2020, Retrieved from: https://khabar.ndtv.com/video/show/news/amit-shah-says-your-vote-decides-that-you-are-with-shaheen-bagh-or-bharat-mata-539129.

12 Ministry of Health and Family Welfare. 2020. 'Update on Novel Coronavirus: One Positive Case Reported in Kerala', PIB, 30 January, https://www.pib.gov.in/PressReleasePage.aspx?PRID=1601095.

13 Ministry of Health and Family Welfare. 2020. 'All Travellers from China Since 15 Jan 2020 Shall be Tested for nCoV', PIB, 30 January, https://www.pib.gov.in/PressReleasePage.aspx?PRID=1601169

14 Ministry of Health and Family Welfare. 2020. 'Update on Novel Coronavirus: One Positive Case Reported in Kerala', PIB, 2 February, https://www.pib.gov.in/PressReleasePage.aspx?PRID=1601625.

15 Ministry of Health and Family Welfare. 2020. 'Update on Novel Coronavirus: Third Positive Case Reported in Kerala', PIB, 3 February, https://www.pib.gov.in/PressReleasePage.aspx?PRID=1601681.

16 Ministry of Health and Family Welfare. 2020. 'High Level Group of Ministers Constituted on Directions of PM

to Review Management of Novel Coronavirus', PIB, 3 February, https://www.pib.gov.in/PressReleasePage.aspx?PRID=1601773

17 Ibid.

18 Lok Sabha Debate. 2020. Seventeenth Series, Third Session, vol. VIII, no. 13, p 23, 5 March, Retrieved from:http://loksabhaph.nic.in/Debates/uncorrecteddebate.aspx.

19 Ibid. p 32.

20 Ibid. p 26.

21 Hardeep Puri Interview in Parliament, 13 March 2020, https://khabar.ndtv.com/video/show/news/steps-have-been-taken-to-deal-with-corona-from-wherever-international-travelers-come-to-india-union-minister-hardeep-puri-543015.

22 Railway Board Chairman Interview in Parliament, 19 March 2020, https://khabar.ndtv.com/video/show/news/railway-board-chairman-appeals-to-people-to-postpone-their-unnecessary-journey-543380.

23 Lala Jha . 2020. 'Mumbai and Delhi Drive Surge in TV Viewership Amid COVID', *Livemint*, 23 April, https://www.livemint.com/industry/media/covid-19-impact-tv-viewership-jumps-driven-by-mumbai-delhi-11587630357318.html.

24 PTI. 2020. '53 Mediapersons Test Coronavirus Positive in Mumbai', *The Hindu*, 20 April, https://www.thehindu.com/news/national/other-states/53-mediapersons-test-coronavirus-positive-in-mumbai/article31388464.ece.

25 Web desk. 2021. '165 Indian Journalists Lost Their Lives to COVID So Far, Says Data', *The Week*, 1 May, https://www.theweek.in/news/india/2021/05/01/165-indian-journalists-have-lost-their-lives-to-covid-so-far-says-data.html,

26 Pallava Bagla. 2020. 'Is India's Communication of COVID Pandemic Running Out of Steam?' *Financial Express*, 12 May, https://www.financialexpress.com/opinion/is-indias-communication-of-covid-pandemic-running-out-of-steam/1955671/.

27 Rohan Venkataramakrishnan. 2020. 'As India's COVID-19 Cases Cross the 100,000 Mark, Why Has Health Ministry Stopped its Briefings?' *Scroll.in.*, 20 May, https://scroll.in/article/962419/as-indias-covid-19-cases-cross-the-100000-mark-why-has-health-ministry-stopped-its-briefings.

28 Press Council of India press release, 10 July 2020, https://presscouncil.nic.in/WriteReadData/Pdf/PressReleaseUPdatedtenjuly.pdf.

29 'Coronavirus: Islamophobia Concerns after India Mosque Outbreak', *BBC*, 3 April 2020, https://www.bbc.com/news/world-asia-india-52147260; Vetticad, Anna M.M. 2020. 'Indian Media Accused of Islamophobia for Its Coronavirus Coverage', *Al Jazeera*, 15 May, https://www.aljazeera.com/news/2020/5/15/indian-media-accused-of-islamophobia-for-its-coronavirus-coverage.

30 Samanwaya Rautray. 2020. 'Demonising Tablighi Jamaat: SC Seeks to Know Mechanism to Deal with Complaints on TV Content', *Economic Times*, 17 November, https://economictimes.indiatimes.com/news/politics-and-nation/sc-not satisfied-with-centres-affidavit-on-pleas-over-tablighi-congregation-media reporting/articleshow/79259347.cms?from=mdr.

31 Express Web Desk, 'Media Reporting of Tablighi Congregation: SC Expresses Displeasure Over Centre's Affidavit', *Indian Express*, 17 November, https://indianexpress.com/article/india/tablighi-jamaat-supreme-court-media-reporting-7054434/.

32 NDTV, 30 May 2020, https://ndtv.in/videos/corona-crisis-hit-msme-sector-badly-550256.

33 NDTV. 30 May 2020, https://ndtv.in/videos/economic-growth-in-shambles-india-gdp-india-economy-550213.

34 Team Inclusion. 2020. 'Mainstreaming the Marginalised', *Inclusion*, 29 May, https://inclusion.in/msme/2020/05/second-national-multi-institutional-survey-on-msmes-in-india/.

35 NDTV, 30 May 2020, https://ndtv.in/videos/corona-crisis-hit-msme-sector-badly-550256.

36 The Hindu Net Desk. 2020. 'Coronavirus updates', *The Hindu*. 26 January, https://www.thehindu.com/news/national/coronavirus-january-26-2021-live-updates/article33664703.ece.

37 Special Correspondent. 2021. 'Coronavirus | India Records More Than 4.14 Lakh New Cases, Over 3,900 Fatalities on May 6, 2021', *The Hindu*, 6 May, https://www.thehindu.

com/news/national/coronavirus-india-records-more-than-414000-new-cases-over-3900-fatalities-on-may-6-2021/article34501680.ece.

38 Federal Emergency Management Agency, https://www.fema.gov/.../economic/funeral-assistance/faq.

39 NDTV, 2 May 2021, https://ndtv.in/videos/delhi-oxygen-crisis-averted-at-madhukar-rainbow-children-hospital-584799.

40 Ministry of Railways. 2021. 'Oxygen Expresses Deliver More Than 32000 MT of LMO to the Nation', PIB, 17 June, https://pib.gov.in/PressReleseDetail.aspx?PRID=1727956.

41 Prime Minister's Office. 2021. '1 Lakh Portable Oxygen Concentrators to be Procured from PM CARES Fund', PM India, 28 April, https://www.pmindia.gov.in/en/news_updates/1-lakh-portable-oxygen-concentrators-to-be-procured-from-pm-cares-fund/?comment=disable.

42 United Nations Office for Disaster Risk Reduction. 2015. 'Sendai Framework for Disaster Risk Reduction 2015–2030', https://www.undrr.org/publication/sendai-framework-disaster-risk-reduction-2015-2030.

CHAPTER 6 AGRICULTURE IN THE TIME OF COVID PANDEMIC

1 Union Agriculture Minister Narendra Singh Tomar's Facebook Post – कोरोनासंक्रमणकीवर्तमानस्थितियोंएवंजागरुकताकोलेकरलाइवसंवाद, https://www.facebook.com/narendrasinghtomarbjp/videos/2581549432164015/.

2 Ministry of Agriculture & Farmers Welfare. 2020. 'Agriculture-Farming and Allied Activities Exempted from Lockdown', PIB, 28 March, https://www.pib.gov.in/PressReleasePage.aspx?PRID=1608785.

3 Ministry of Agriculture & Farmers Welfare. 2020. 'Govt Gives Benefits to Farmers on Crop Loan Repayments Due to COVID-19 lockdown', PIB, 30 March, https://pib.gov.in/PressReleasePage.aspx?PRID=1609282.

4 Ministry of Agriculture & Farmers Welfare. 2020. 'In wake of COVID-19 spread, ICAR issues Advisory to Farmers for Rabi Crops', PIB, 30 March, https://www.pib.gov.in/PressReleasePage.aspx?PRID=1609604.

5 Ministry of Agriculture & Farmers Welfare. 2020. 'More Lockdown Relaxations for Agriculture-Farming Sector', PIB. 4 April, https://www.pib.gov.in/PressReleasePage.aspx?PRID=1611035.

6 Ministry of Micro, Small and Medium Enterprises. Annual Report: 2018–2019.

7 Vyas, Mahesh. 2020. 'Unemployment Rate Over 23%', Centre for Monitoring Indian Economy, 7 April 2020.

8 Ministry of Agriculture & Farmers Welfare. 2020. 'Shri Narendra Singh Tomar Chairs Meeting with State Agriculture Ministers to review relief steps for farmers', PIB. 9 April, https://www.pib.gov.in/PressReleasePage.aspx?PRID=1612410.

9 'There Is No Dearth of Fruits and Vegetables in the Country: Agriculture Minister', NDTV, 10 April 2020. https://khabar.ndtv.com/video/show/news/there-is-no-dearth-of-fruits-and-vegetables-in-the-country-union-agriculture-minister-545283.

10 Prime Minister's Office. 2020. 'PM Interacts with CMs to Strategize Ahead for Tackling COVID-19', PIB, 11 April, https://www.pib.gov.in/PressReleasePage.aspx?PRID=1613317.

11 Ministry of Agriculture & Farmers Welfare. 2020. 'Overcoming Lockdown Restrictions, Sowing of Summer Crops Continues Uninterrupted', PIB, 11 April, https://www.pib.gov.in/PressReleasePage.aspx?PRID=1613342.

12 Ministry of Agriculture & Farmers Welfare. 2020. 'Government Initiates Dialogue to Resurrect Agri Sector Exports in the Aftermath of Current COVID-19 Crisis', PIB, 14 April,. https://pib.gov.in/PressReleaseIframePage.aspx?PRID=1614278#.XpV5bgioZM4.whatsapp.

13 Ministry of Agriculture & Farmers Welfare. 2020. 'Union Agriculture Minister Chairs the National Conference on Kharif Crops 2020 through Video Conference', PIB, 16 April, https://www.pib.gov.in/PressReleasePage.aspx?PRID=1614994

14 'In Last One Week Unemployment Rate Reached upto 23.4%', NDTV, 8 April2020, from: https://khabar.ndtv.com/video/show/news/in-last-one-week-unemployment-rate-reached-upto-23-4-percent-545063.

15 'Ram Vilas Paswan Says States Should Help with National Disaster Relief Fund', NDTV, 13 April 2020, https://khabar.

ndtv.com/video/show/news/ram-vilas-paswan-saysstate-should-help-with-national-disaster-relief-fund-545554.

16 Reserve Bank of India Governor Statement. 17 April 2020, https://rbidocs.rbi.org.in/rdocs/Content/PDFs/GOVERNORSTATEMENTF22E618703AE48A4B2F6E-C4A8003F88D.PDF.

17 Radheshyam Jadhav 2020. 'Covid-19 impact: Dabbawalas Turn to Agriculture for Survival', *The Hindu BusinessLine*, 17 July, https://www.thehindubusinessline.com/news/variety/covid-19-impact-dabbawalas-turn-to-agriculture-for-survival/article32112328.ece.

18 Prime Minister's Office. 2020. 'English Rendering of Prime Minister Shri Narendra Modi's Address to the Nation on 12.5.2020', PIB, 12 May, https://pib.gov.in/PressReleasePage.aspx?PRID=1623418

19 'Census Reports 1921', Office of the Registrar General and Census Commissioner, India, https://censusindia.gov.in/Census_And_You/old_report/census_1921.aspx.

20 Ibid.

21 Siddharth Chandra and Eva Kassens-Noor. 2014. 'The Evolution of Pandemic Influenza: Evidence from India, 1918–19', *BMC Infectious Diseases*, Vol. 14. Article no. 510,47, https://bmcinfectdis.biomedcentral.com/articles/10.1186/1471-2334-14-510.

22 'Census Reports 1921', Office of the Registrar General and Census Commissioner, India, https://censusindia.gov.in/Census_And_You/old_report/census_1921.aspx

23 'Census Reports 1921', Office of the Registrar General and Census Commissioner, India, https://censusindia.gov.in/Census_And_You/old_report/census_1921.aspx.

24 Sachin P. Mampatta. 2020. 'How Long Did India's Per Capita GDP Take to Recover after 1918 Pandemic?' *Business Standard*, 12 June, https://www.business-standard.com/article/economy-policy/how-long-did-india-s-per-capita-gdp-take-to-recover-after-1918-pandemic-120061200351_1.html.

25 'Census Reports 1921', Office of the Registrar General and Census Commissioner, India, https://censusindia.gov.in/Census_And_You/old_report/census_1921.aspx.

26 Saeed Khan. 2020. '1918 Spanish Flu Cure Ordered by Doctors Was Contraindicated in Gandhiji's principles', *Times of India*, 14 April,

https://timesofindia.indiatimes.com/city/ahmedabad/1918-spanish-flu-cure-ordered-by-docs-was-contraindicated-in-gandhijis-principles/articleshow/75130706.cms.

27 Catharine Arnold. *Pandemic 1918: The Story of the Deadliest Influenza in History*. London: Michael O'Mara Books Limited, 2018.

28 Patt Morrison. 2020. 'What the Deadly 1918 Flu Epidemic Can Teach Us about Our Coronavirus Reaction', *Los Angeles Times*. 11 March, https://www.latimes.com/opinion/story/2020-03-11/1918-flu-epidemic-coronavirus.

29 Thomas Weber and Dennis Dalton. 2020. 'Gandhi and the Pandemic', *Economic and Political Weekly*, Vol. 55, Issue no. 25, 20 June. , 2020.

30 Reserve Bank of India. Governor's Statement. May 22, 2020. Page-4. Retrieved from: https://rbidocs.rbi.org.in/rdocsContent/PDFs/GOVERNORSTA1BE078EC-8D2F4F53A8C3A74AE98E4573.PDF

31 Cabinet. 2020. 'PM Chairs Cabinet Meeting to Give Historic Boost to Rural India', PIB, 3 June, https://pib.gov.in/PressReleasePage.aspx?PRID=1629033.

32 'Are Dynamic Shifts Underway in the Indian Economy?' Shaktikanta Das, RBI Governor, Address to CII National Council, Mumbai, *Reserve Bank of India*, 27 July 2020, https://www.rbi.org.in/Scripts/BS_SpeechesView.aspx?Id=1098

33 Prime Minister's Office. 2020. 'PM Launches Financing Facility of ₹1 Lakh Crore Under Agriculture Infrastructure Fund', PIB, 9 August, https://www.pib.gov.in/PressReleasePage.aspx?PRID=1644529.

34 Geeta Pandey. 2021. 'Covid-19: India's Holiest River Is Swollen with Bodies', *BBC*, 19 May, https://www.bbc.com/news/world-asia-india-57154564.

35 Ibid.

36 https://www.allstudyjournal.com/article/544/3-2-12-338.pdf

37 NDTV, 14 May 2021, https://ndtv.in/videos/pm-narendra-modi-over-coronavirus-spreading-in-villages-586172.

38 Prime Minister's Office. 2021. 'PM Chairs a High Level Meeting on Covid and Vaccination-Related Situation', PIB, 15 May, https://www.pib.gov.in/PressReleasePage.aspx?PRID=1718787.

39 'SOP on COVID-19 Containment & Management in Peri-urban, Rural & Tribal Areas', Ministry of Health Affairs, 16 May 2021, https://www.mohfw.gov.in/pdf/SOPonCOVID-19Containment&ManagementinPeriurbanRural&tribalareas.pdf.

40 'PM Chokes Up As He Pays Tribute: "This Virus Took Away Many Loved Ones"', NDTV, 21 May 2021, https://www.ndtv.com/india-news/pm-narendra-modi-chokes-up-as-he-pays-tribute-this-virus-took-away-many-loved-ones-2446388.

41 'State of Working India 2021 Report', Axim Premji University, 5 May 2021, https://cse.azimpremjiuniversity.edu.in/state-of-working-india/swi-2021/.

42 Himanshu Shekhar Mishra. 2021. 'In the Second Wave of Corona, 70 Lakh People Lost Their Jobs in India', NDTV, 4 May, https://ndtv.in/india-news/covid-19-second-wave-left-another-7-million-people-jobless-in-april-2428039

43 Himanshu Shekhar Mishra . 2021. 'Impact of Corona Crisis and Lockdown on MSME Sector, Garment Producers in Serious Financial Crisis', NDTV, 10 May, https://ndtv.in/india-news/covid-crisis-and-lockdown-impact-on-msme-sector-garment-manufacturers-face-huge-financial-crisis-2439057.

44 'Unemployment Rate in India', Centre for Monitoring Indian Economy, https://unemploymentinindia.cmie.com/kommon/bin/sr.php?kall=wshowtab&tabno=0002.

45 'Lockdown Fallout: Impact on Migrant Workers', NDTV, 23 May 2021, https://www.ndtv.com/video/news/news/covid-19-lockdown-lockdown-fallout-impact-on-migrant-workers-587306; https://ndtv.in/videos/effect-of-lockdown-villagers-face-economic-crisis-mnrega-work-in-lockdown-586968

CHAPTER 7 MIGRATION AND FOOD SECURITY DURING THE PANDEMIC

1 '"Black fungus" declared an epidemic in 4 states, 1 UT', *Times of India*, 21 May 2021, https://timesofindia.indiatimes.com/india/black-fungus-declared-an-epidemic-in-4-states-1-ut/articleshow/82804720.cms.

2 BBC News, 20 May 2020, https://www.bbc.com/news/world-asia-india-52672764

3 India Today Web Desk. 2020. 'Pregnant Migrant Labourer Delivers Baby while Walking Home, Walks Another 150 Km after Delivery', *India Today*, 13 May, https://www.indiatoday.in/india/story/pregnant-migrant-labourer-delivers-baby-while-walking-home-1677374-2020-05-13; 'Pregnant Migrant Labourer Delivers Baby while Walking Home amid COVID-19 Lockdown', *Zee News* 13 May 2020, https://zeenews.india.com/video/india/pregnant-migrant-labourer-delivers-baby-while-walking-home-amid-covid-19-lockdown-2283321.html.

4 Manisha Priyam and Mridusmita Bordoloi. 2020. 'Documenting the Story of India's Migrant Distress', *Hindustan Times*, 29 May, https://www.hindustantimes.com/analysis/documenting-the-story-of-india-s-migrant-distress/story-sVC8sCHFetXYBPKLa1OhZM.html.

5 Express News Service. 2020. 'West Bengal Migrant Labourers Who Returned to Village Quarantine Themselves on Tree Branches', *New Indian Express*, 29 March, https://www.newindianexpress.com/nation/2020/mar/28/west-bengal-migrant-labourers-who-returned-to-village-quarantine-themselves-on-banyan-tree-branches-2122629.html.

6 PTI. 2020. '29% of Migrant Workers Have Returned to Cities while 45% Want to Return', *Mint*, 3 August, https://www.livemint.com/news/india/29-of-migrant-workers-have-returned-to-cities-while-45-want-to-return-survey-11596447935032.html.

7 Arun Kumar. 2021. 'Is the Latest Change in India's Vaccination Policy the Final Twist in the Tale?' *The Wire*, 11 June, https://thewire.in/government/is-the-latest-change-in-indias-vaccination-policy-the-final-twist-in-the-tale.

8 'Migrant Labour Welfare: Supreme Court Orders Rations without ID Proof, Community Kitchens, Transport (Read Order)', *India Legal*, 13 May 2021, https://www.indialegallive.com/constitutional-law-news/supreme-court-news/migrant-labour-lockdown-ration-no-aadhaar/.

9 Shreehari Paliath. 2021.'Savings Dry Up, Few Jobs: Covid Second Wave Hits Migrant Workers Harder', *Business Standard*, 1 June, https://www.business-standard.com/article/current-affairs/migrant-workers-hit-harder-by-second-wave-as-savings-dry-up-scanty-jobs-121060100140_1.html.

10 International Organization for Migration, 2019, 132.
11 Ministry of Housing and Urban Poverty Alleviation,'Report of the Working Group on Migration', 3.
12 KNOMAD. 2020,5.
13 KNOMAD. 2020, 6.
14 Ministry of Finance.Government of India, 2019.Vol. 1.199–200.
15 Piu Mukherjee, Paul G. D. Bino, J.I. Pathan. 'Migrant Workers in Informal Sector: A Probe into Working Conditions', ATLMRI Discussion Paper Series Discussion Paper 9, p. 5 (n.d.), http://www.shram.org/uploadFiles/20130305105845.pdf
16 Harriss-White et al., 2014, 39.
17 *Down to Earth*. 12 July 2020.
18 Prashantand Jha and Ishita Mishra. 2020. 'Uttarakhand's "Ghost Villages" Spring Back to Life', *Times of India*, 17 June, https://timesofindia.indiatimes.com/city/dehradun/uttarakhands-ghost-villages-spring-back-to-life/articleshow/76412902.cms; Upadhyay, Kavita. 2018. 'Inside the Ghost Villages of Uttarakhand', *Indian Express*, 24 June, https://indianexpress.com/article/india/uttarakhand-baluni-saina-bhootiya-abandoned-villages-migration-5230715/.
19 'Unemployment Rate in India', *CMIE*, https://unemploymentinindia.cmie.com/kommon/bin/sr.php?kall=wsttimeseries&index_code=050050000000&dtype=total.
20 Sunil Prabhu. 2020. 'No Data on Migrant Deaths, So No Compensation: Government to Parliament', NDTV, 15 September, https://www.ndtv.com/india-news/no-data-on-migrant-deaths-so-no-compensation-government-to-parliament-2295409.
21 Anisha Dutta. 2020. '198 Migrant Workers Killed in Road Accidents during Lockdown: Report', *Hindustan Times*, 2 June, https://www.hindustantimes.com/india-news/198-migrant-workers-killed-in-road-accidents-during-lockdown-report/story-hTWzAWMYnokyycKw1dyKqL.html.
22 'One Nation, One Ration Card System: List of 17 States which Have Completed Implementation', *Hindustan Times*, 11 March 2021, https://www.hindustantimes.com/india-news/one-nation-one-ration-card-system-list-of-17-states-which-have-completed-implementation-101615477779670.html.

23 PTI. 2021. 'SC Asks States, UTs to Implement "One Nation, One Ration Card' Scheme",*Times of India*, 11 June, https://timesofindia.indiatimes.com/india/sc-asks-states-uts-to-implement-one-nation-one-ration-card-scheme/articleshow/83436198.cms.

24 Arvind Narrain. 2021. 'States Have to Ensure Food Security for the Marginalised in the Pandemic', *News Minute*, 21 May, https://www.thenewsminute.com/article/states-have-ensure-food-security-marginalised-pandemic-149261.

25 'The State of Food Security and the Nutrition of the World 2020'. Food and Agricultural Organization, 4.

26 Ibid.

27 'Pocket Book of Agricultural Statistics 2017', Directorate of Economics and Statistics, Ministry of Agriculture and Farmers Welfare, 2017, 2, https://agricoop.nic.in/sites/default/files/pocketbook_0.pdf.

28 Ibid., 20.

29 PTI. 2020. 'India's Foodgrains Production to Touch Record 295.67 MT in 2019-20 Crop Year', *Financial Express*, 15 May, https://www.financialexpress.com/economy/indias-foodgrains-production-to-touch-record-295-67-mt-in-2019-20-crop-year/1960151/; 'Bumper Harvest: Foodgrains Output to touch 296 mt in 2019-20',*The Hindu Business Line*, 15 May 2020, https://www.thehindubusinessline.com/economy/agri-business/foodgrain-output-likely-to-be-at-296-million-tonnes-for-2019-20-3rd-advance-estimates/article31591886.ece.

30 Mausami Singh. 2020. 'Raped in Chitrakoot: Minor girls Forced to Trade Bodies for ₹150-200 Daily during Lockdown', *India Today*, 8 July, https://www.indiatoday.in/india/story/raped-in-chitrakoot-minor-girls-forced-to-trade-bodies-for-rs-150-200-daily-during-lockdown-1698173-2020-07-08.

31 Ibid.

32 Food and Public Distribution Ministry, Government of India, 2 July 2020.

33 'Evaluation Study on Role of Public Distribution System in Shaping Household and Nutritional Security India', NITI Aayog, Government of India, December 2016, IV.DMEO, Report No. 233. New Delhi. https://niti.gov.in/writereaddata/

files/document_publication/Final%20PDS%20Report-new.pdf.

34 'NGO Points Out "Exclusion Errors" in PDS', *The Hindu*, 2 August 2018, https://www.thehindu.com/news/national/other-states/ngo-points-out-exclusion-errors-in-pds/article24576686.ece.

35 Ibid.

36 Bram Spruyt, et al. 2016, 2.

37 Noel Semple. 2020.

38 Ibid.

39 Mathur, 2013, 2.

40 Moushumi Das Gupta. 2019. 'Why Modi has created a new "super power centre" in his PMO', *The Print*, 13 June, https://theprint.in/india/governance/why-modi-has-created-a-new-super-power-centre-in-his-pmo/249446/.

41 Lowi, 1972, 308.

CHAPTER 8 UNPREDICTABLE LIVES AND LIVELIHOOD WITH COVID-19

1 The Wire Staff. 2020. 'India's GDP Growth Drops to 5% for First Quarter of FY20, Slowest in Six Years', *The Wire*, 30 August, https://thewire.in/economy/india-gdp-growth-slows-5-q1-fy20.

2 'Quotable quotes by John Kenneth Galbraith', Goodreads.com.

3 'World Economic Situation And Prospects: August 2020 Briefing, No. 140', UN, 3 August 2020, https://www.un.org/development/desa/dpad/publication/world-economic-situation-and-prospects-august-2020-briefing-no-140/.

4 Udit Misra. 2020. 'India GDP Growth Contracts 23.9%: What Is the Economics behind the Math?' *Indian Express*, 6 September, https://indianexpress.com/article/explained/gdp-contraction-23-9-the-economics-behind-the-math-6578046/?utm_source=newzmate&utm_medium=email&utm_campaign=explained&tqid=1.SmfnI_D1YBeK3thT3MUF4l9srpvMyiJi33ITVZ.w.

5 'Building Atmanirbhar Bharat & Overcoming COVID-19', *India.gov.in*, https://www.india.gov.in/spotlight/building-atmanirbhar-bharat-overcoming-covid-19.

6 '229th Report on Management of COVID-19 Pandemic Related Issues', Department Related Parliamentary Standing Committee on Home Affairs, Rajya Sabha Secretariat, New Delhi, 21 December 2020, 49.

7 Aanchal Magazine. 2020. 'Breaking Down GST: Slabs, Payments, Dispute', *Indian Express*, 13 August, https://indianexpress.com/article/explained/breaking-down-gst-slabs-payments-dispute-6549353/.

8 ETHealthWorld. 2020. 'Managing Public Health during COVID-19', *Economic Times*, 19 May, https://health.economictimes.indiatimes.com/news/industry/managing-public-health-during-covid-19/75826907.

9 Christophe Jaffrelot and Utsav Shah. 2020. 'India Needs to Urgently Step into the Domain of Healthcare', *Indian Express*, 9 June, https://indianexpress.com/article/opinion/columns/coronavirus-epidemic-healthcare-system-public-hospitals-6449264/.

10 Ibid.

11 MD Bureau. 2020. '0.55 Govt Beds Per 1,000 Population: Report Flags Low Govt Hospital Bed Availability in India', Medical Dialogues, 25 March, https://medicaldialogues.in/category/latest-news/055-govt-beds-per-1000-population-report-flags-low-govt-hospital-bed-availability-in-india-64226.

12 ETHealthWorld. 2020. 'Managing Public Health during COVID-19', *Economic Times*, 19 May, https://health.economictimes.indiatimes.com/news/industry/managing-public-health-during-covid-19/75826907.

13 'Policy Brief: COVID-19 and the Need for Action on Mental Health', UN, 13 May 2020, https://www.un.org/sites/un2.un.org/files/un_policy_brief-covid_and_mental_health_final.pdf.

14 '229th Report on Management of COVID-19 Pandemic Related Issues', Department Related Parliamentary Standing Committee on Home Affairs, 21 December 2020, 43.

15 A. S. Wharton. 2006. *The Sociology of Gender*. New Jersey: Wiley-Blackwell Publishers.

16 Deeptiman Tiwary. 2021. 'Domestic Violence, Trafficking Rose in lockdown: House Panel', *Indian Express*, 16 March,

https://indianexpress.com/article/india/domestic-violence-trafficking-lockdown-7230112/.

17 Atul Thakur. 2020. 'Why Umemployment Rate Is Falling in Some States but Rising in Others', *Times of India*, https://timesofindia.indiatimes.com/india/why-unemployment-rate-is-falling-in-some-states-but-rising-in-others/articleshow/76148653.cms.

18 Koustav Das. 2020. 'Coronavirus: 5 Indian Sectors that Need Urgent Help as Virus Ravages Economy', *India Today*, 23 April, https://www.indiatoday.in/business/story/coronavirus-5-indian-sectors-that-need-urgent-help-as-virus-ravages-economy-1670099-2020-04-23.

19 Sarah Steingruber et al. March 2020, 'Corruption in the Time of COVID-19: A Double Threat for Low-income Countries', Anti-Corruption Resource Centre, https://www.u4.no/publications/corruption-in-the-time-of-covid-19-a-double-threat-for-low-income-countries.

20 Venkatesha Babu. 2020. 'Siddaramaiah Alleges Corruption of ₹2,200 Crore on Govt's Purchase of Covid-19 Equipment', *Hindustan Times*, 3 July, https://www.hindustantimes.com/india-news/siddaramaiah-alleges-corruption-of-rs-2-200-crore-on-govt-s-purchase-of-covid-19-equipment/story-5TLUvDFK7buzUOAiSzOuoL.html.

21 HT Correspondents. 2021. 'Record Corruption in the Name of Handling Covid in Maharashtra, Alleges Fadnavis', MSN, 2 March, https://www.msn.com/en-in/news/other/record-corruption-in-the-name-of-handling-covid-in-maharashtra-alleges-fadnavis/ar-BB1eai7X.

22 'PM inaugurates Zen Garden and Kaizen Academy at AMA, Ahmedabad', PMIndia,gov.in, 27 June 2021, https://www.pmindia.gov.in/en/news_updates/pm-inaugurates-zen-garden-and-kaizen-academy-at-ama-ahmedabad/?comment=disable.

CHAPTER 9 EDUCATION FOR EDUCATION

1 Himanshu Shekhar Mishra. 2021. 'Use Satellite TV To Beam Classes For Poor Students Amid Covid: Parliamentary Panel To Centre', NDTV, 21 June, https://www.ndtv.com/india-

news/use-satellite-tv-to-beam-classes-for-poor-students-amid-covid-parliamentary-panel-to-centre-2469128.

CONCLUSION

1 'Coronavirus May 8, 2021: 53,605 New Cases in Maharashtra; US CDC Acknowledges Virus is Airborne', *India Today*, 9 May 2021, https://www.indiatoday.in/india/story/india-coronavirus-live-news-updates-covid-death-toll-covid-19-vaccine-drive-1800142-2021-05-08.
2 Worldometer, 28 June 2021, https://www.worldometers.info/coronavirus/.
3 Utkarsh Kumar. 2021. 'IPL 2021 Suspended Amid Rising Number of Covid-19 Cases among Players and Support Staff', *India Today*, 4 May, 2021. https://www.indiatoday.in/sports/ipl-2021/story/ipl-2021-suspended-amid-rising-number-of-covid-19-cases-among-players-and-support-staff-1798678-2021-05-04.
4 Soutik Biswas. 2021. 'Covid-19: Has India's Deadly Second Wave Peaked?', 26 May, https://www.bbc.com/news/world-asia-india-57225922.
5 *Economic Survey 2020–2021*, Vol. II, 47.
6 *Monthly Economic Review*, February 2021. Department of Economic Affairs, Ministry of Finance, 1.
7 *Monthly Economic Review*, February 2021. Department of Economic Affairs, Ministry of Finance,6–7.

APPENDIX

1 The Constitution of India. Government of India, 2019. Ministry of Law and Justice, New Delhi.
2 This doctrine is not dependent on any constitutional provisions or presence of any legislative enactment. We find evidence of state obligation to protect its citizens in the Famine Relief Code adopted after the Great Famine of 1876–1878. This famine leads to the constitution of the Famine Commission of 1880 and eventual adoption of the Famine Relief Code. India probably has the world's oldest disaster relief code, which was put in

place in 1880. This relief code provides details of the relief to be given by the government to the affected people.

National Institute of Disaster Management, 2015. Handbook on Disaster Management for Nodal Officers (Compilation). Ministry of Home Affairs, Government of India, New Delhi, page 12.

3 State Disaster Management Plans. Retrieved from: http://nidm.gov.in on 25 June 2020

4 National Institute of Disaster Management, 2015. Disaster Management Act, 2005. Page 100.

5 Ibid

6 Epidemic Diseases (Amendment) Ordinance, 2020. Retrieved from https://dashamlav.com/epidemic-disease-act-1897/ on 23 June 2020.

7 NDMA Vision. Retrieved from: https://ndma.gov.in/en/about-ndma/vision.html on 1 July 2020.

8 Main Pillars of National Policy on Disaster Management. Retrieved from: https://ndma.gov.in/images/policyplan/dmplan/ndmp-2019.pdf on 23 June 2020.

9 Ibid.

INDEX

ABOUT THE AUTHORS

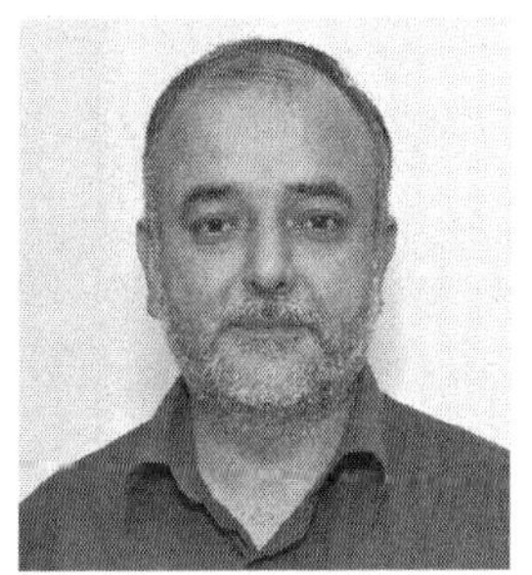

Vinay Sharma: Reflexivity, spirituality, market opportunity development, the Ganga, Himalaya and forest are the keywords encompassing Professor Vinay Sharma from the Indian Institute of Technology (IIT), Roorkee. He has been teaching innovation, strategy, marketing communication and product and brand management along with pursuing projects on developing a value chain for establishing pine needles as a source of household energy and generating livelihood in the Himalayas. Supported by an eminent group of academicians and zealous scholars, he has contributed in several doctoral researches, research papers and books. Healthcare to the rural population, ancient development models, low-cost energy and the purpose of management education (which is also the subject of his book *Masters Speak on Management Education in India*, published by Bloomsbury India) have been his areas of concern while affordability and profitability have been the premise of his research engagements.

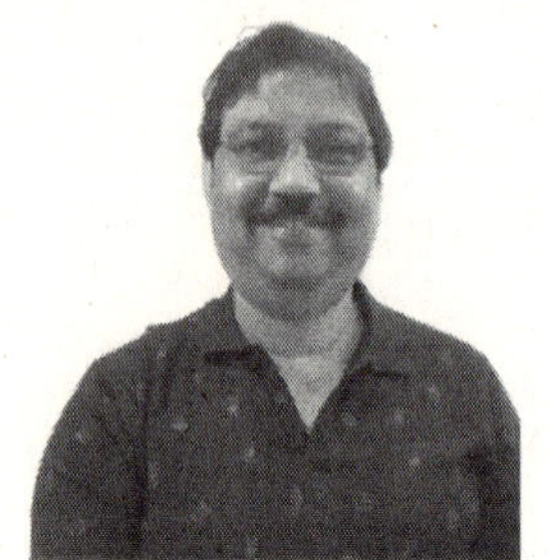

Rabindranath Bhattacharyya is currently a professor of political science at the University of Burdwan, West Bengal. His research area focuses on democratic governance with special focus on poverty alleviation and disaster management across countries. He was appointed the Australia Awards Ambassador for the year 2014–2015 by the Australian High Commissioner to India. He has been awarded the Australian Government Endeavour Post-Doctoral Research Award, 2009, and the AIC Australian Studies (Senior) Visiting Fellowship 2007–2008 for visiting five universities in Australia. He has co-edited three books and has a number of papers and book chapters published in both national and international journals and books. He has presented papers and chaired sessions at national and international conferences and seminars spreading over eight countries. He has successfully supervised PhD theses of six candidates from India and Bangladesh and acted as PhD examiner of various universities within and outside India. He has also acted as an expert for UPSC, SPSC, West Bengal College Service Commission and different state universities in India in various capacities.

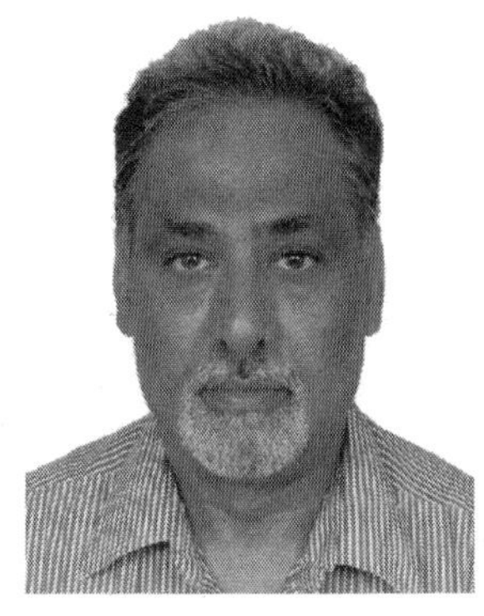

Sanjeev Kumar Mahajan, PhD, is a professor of public administration at Himachal Pradesh University, Shimla. He was awarded the Panjab University gold medal and the Best Teacher Award for 2021 by Himachal Pradesh University. He has presented research articles at national and international conferences. He has more than 50 publications, including four books published in India and research articles worldwide. Two edited books have been published by Business Expert Press, New York.

He has held various important administrative positions. Recently, he was appointed on the board of directors of the Asian Association of Public Administration and is also the vice president of the Indian Public Administration Association. He was a visiting fellow for the University Grants Commission under the Indo-Hungary Cultural Exchange Program. He was also an external peer reviewer as an overseas QA expert for universities in Bangladesh.

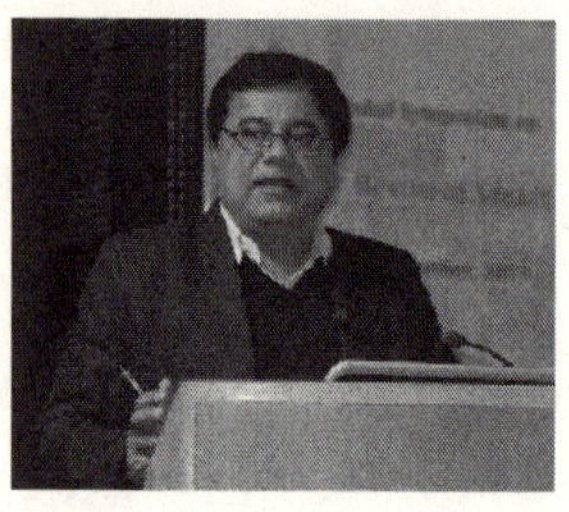

Himanshu Shekhar Mishra works as senior editor (political & current affairs) at New Delhi Television (NDTV). He was part of the prime minister's official entourage to United Nations' Annual Session in New York (September 2003) and the Indo-Turkish Summit held in Ankara and Istanbul (2003). He has covered the prime minister's official visits to Pakistan (January 2004) and Afghanistan (August 2005) as a TV news journalist. He has also reported and researched on climate-related disasters, legal rights of disaster victims, threats posed by climate change to sustainable development and disaster journalism.

His paper on the unprecedented floods in Jammu and Kashmir in September 2014 was selected for presentation at the 3rd United Nations World Conference on Disaster Risk Reduction held in Sendai, Japan, in March 2015. Till date, he has five published research papers in international volumes on disaster management. He holds a Master of Philosophy degree from the Centre for West Asian Studies, Jawaharlal Nehru University, New Delhi. He did his post-graduation in political science from JNU (1995–1997).